Trois taches de couleur sur un plan d'Orléans...

Le lourd épais sac à dos était resté là des mois après la mort de Khaled.

Hier, je l'ai ouvert enfin.

Plein de papiers administratifs — De la main de Khaled : des listes d'adresses ou de téléphones en arabe, et des exercices d'écriture.

Ce plan, pourquoi l'avait-il gardé alors qu'après huit années vécues à la maison il connaissait la ville peut-être mieux que moi ?

La tache verte, c'est en face de la gare, L'Office français de l'immigration.

La tache rouge, c'est la Poste centrale (et la place où, presque toujours, "des noirs, africains — probablement — (pas mal de femmes, des enfants poursuivant les pigeons) sont rassemblés, par petits groupes..." — Papiers !).

La tache jaune, c'est la maison (ou la rue : les tracés ont fondu dans la couleur).

Il n'y a pas de tache sur les bords ou îles de la Loire où il cherchait refuge avant de vivre avec nous.

Three spots of color on a map of Orléans…

The thick heavy knapsack had been sitting there for months after Khaled's death.

Yesterday, I finally opened it.

Full of administrative papers — Written in Khaled's hand: lists of addresses or telephone numbers in Arabic, and writing exercises.

This map, why had he kept it since after eight years in our house he knew the city perhaps better than I did?

The green spot is the French Immigration Office, in front of the train station.

The red spot is the Central Post Office (and the square where, at any time almost, "Blacks, Africans — probably — (quite a few women, children chasing pigeons) are assembled, in small groups…" — Papers!).

The yellow spot is the house (or the street: the color has blurred the outlines).

There is no spot on the banks or the islands of the Loire where he looked for shelter before coming to live with us.

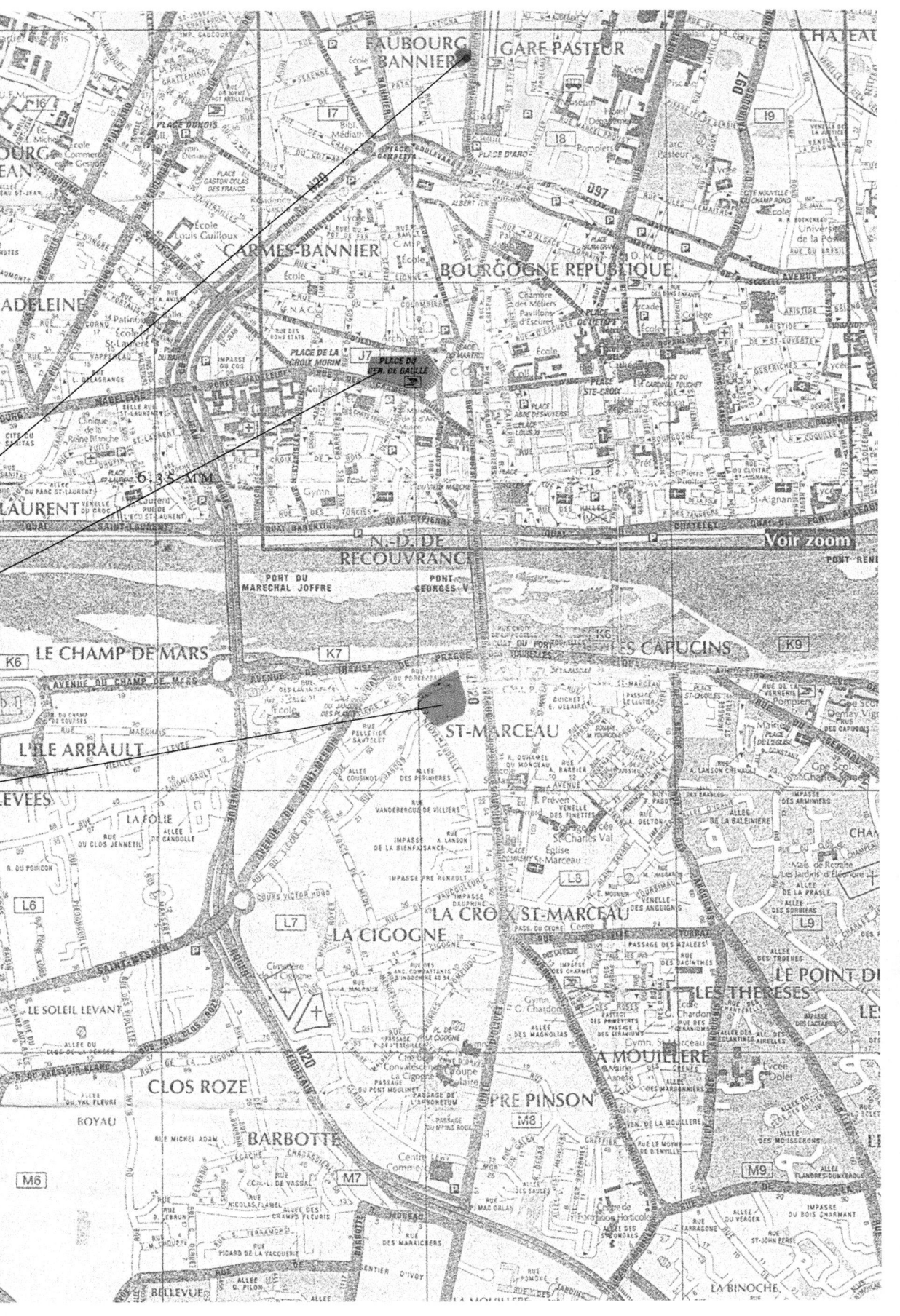

CLAUDE MOUCHARD

Entangled Papers! Notes

Translated and with an Introduction by

MARY SHAW

Preface by

MICHEL DEGUY

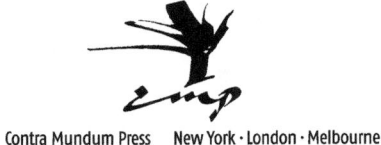

Contra Mundum Press · New York · London · Melbourne

Entangled — Papers! — Notes
© 2017 Claude Mouchard;
translation © 2017 Mary Shaw

First Contra Mundum Press
edition 2017.

All Rights Reserved under
International & Pan-American
Copyright Conventions.
No part of this book may be
reproduced in any form or by
any electronic means, including
information storage and retrieval
systems, without permission in
writing from the publisher,
except by a reviewer who may
quote brief passages in a review.

Library of Congress
Cataloguing-in-Publication Data
Mouchard, Claude, 1941–

[Entangled, — Papers! — Notes.
English.]

Entangled, — Papers! — Notes /
Claude Mouchard;
Translated from the French by
Mary Shaw.

—1st Contra Mundum Press
Edition
296 pp., 7 x 10 in.

ISBN 9781940625256

   I. Mouchard, Claude.
  II. Title.
 III. Shaw, Mary.
 IV. Translator & Introduction.
  V. Deguy, Michel.
 VI. Preface.
VII. Segalini, Alessandro.
VIII. Calligraphy (title).

2017947794

Table of Contents

o	PREFACE · *The Unrealizable*, by Michel Deguy
x	INTRODUCTION
xxx	ACKNOWLEDGEMENTS
o	*Entangled*
22	*Papers!*
56	*Notes*
58	From Darfur to the Loire [...]
72	"& whether this is living?"
82	Perpetual dawn?
94	Alone, Khaled?
122	*Enchevêtrée*
144	*Papiers!*
178	*Notes*
180	Du Darfour à la Loire [...]
194	« & si c'est cela vivre ? »
204	Aube perpétuelle ?
216	Tout seul, Khaled ?

Preface

The Unrealizable

Mary Shaw catches and isolates the term that condenses, for Claude Mouchard, the great task, responsibility, and program of the writer as "witness of his time": *realize*.

> "What am I trying to do with such sentences?
> 'Realize' is the expression that comes to me."[1]

How does one "realize"?

It's a more than common word, very colloquial and "simple," even if one were to tell Mr. Jourdain, who uses it, that he is philosophizing unwittingly.[2] It belongs to ordinary, non-philosophical prose, even though it comes from philosophy, and — fatally, I was about to say — refers back to it. The *sentences* (as your basic Wittgensteinian would put it) that are most inclined to perform it are negative ones. "Ah! I *hadn't realized* that [...]!" — and here I am, in the process of "realizing"... I cite the word's occurrences (no negation here: "dare to **realize**," "in order to realize"[3]) in the *Notes* (which I am not characterizing, so as not to fall into facile hyperbolic praise) recording eight years of extraordinary hospitality: they retrace tirelessly, without measure, in what manner and to what *end* Claude Mouchard *realizes* (becomes fully aware *and* gives a full account of) what happens — happens to him, happens to those he hosts. To *note* and to *departition* are the experience's decisive terms.

As a near-synonym of "realizing," common usage often speaks of "translating." How does one translate lived experience? The first use of this verb in fact refers less to the commerce among foreign languages than to "expressing oneself." "Translate" emotions, "render" them, is what is asked of the artist. The carrying of experience from one incarnated subjectivity over to another, above the abyss

---

1   See Introduction, page XIII.
2   In Molière's *Le Bourgeois gentilhomme* (*The Bourgeois Gentleman*, II, IV), Mr. Jourdain learns from his philosophy teacher that he has used prose all his life, without being aware of it. Translator's note [TN].
3   See *Notes*, pages 112, 114.

of alterity; a leap that is marked, as is always the case in our language, by the *trans* and the *meta*. The trance of the *trans* is the work of the artist — but first that of any speaking being who strives to relate and persuade.

This is not the place to "critique" this tireless expectation-and-demand of the public (of the us-all) on its artists; this perennial, intense, intolerable expression of the quest for expressivity (for the *well-rendered*) that presupposes the "abyssal" difference within "me" between the inside (*interior intimo meo*)[4] and the outside; and the separation between a subject and an *other*, an absolutely exterior alter ego.

How does one make whatever is written by moved (yet mastered) thinking pass through the body ("the affections of the human body," a Spinozian would say)? Not just fight against insensitivity by alerting listeners and readers to the growing general horror (growing in "generalization," triggering an "all of mankind" than can be aware of it), to "all the misery in the world," which we recognize while being *in*capable of "taking it in" (Michel Rocard),[5] to the ongoing hominicide; but also bear witness to one, for one, this one, this infinitely near and infinitely other being at the edge of my consciousness: neither "the other" in general, nor my "Christian" neighbor.

Finally, and anxiously: what is it to bear witness?

In an expert and breathless, spasmodic and virtuosic transposition mobilizing typographical tools to translate tones like the *neumes* of his prose,[6] Mouchard bears witness to and for the existence of Khaled.[7] Khaled has lived. Transposition of tonalities: the soliloquy, the vociferation, the ongoing process of "realizing"; staging, for a reader's eyes, of a score of pensive emotions.

---

4   St. Augustine, *Confessions*, III, 6.11. [TN]

5   The French socialist Prime Minister Michel Rocard famously said, in a 1989 speech about immigration policy, that France could not welcome "all the misery in the world." [TN]

6   I was reading Jean-Claude Schmitt's beautiful book. One finds there (finally) a clarification of *neumes*: "Neumes do not transcribe sounds, they *express* their movement and oscillations. […] Neumes are not prescriptive, but indicative." See *Les Rythmes au Moyen Âge* (Paris: Gallimard, 2016) 77 ff.

7   The last of the *Notes* series in this volume, "Alone, Khaled?" («Tout seul, Khaled?»), responds to the untimely death of Khaled Mahjoub Mansour, a refugee from Darfur who lived in Claude Mouchard's house for eight years. [TN]

Claude bears witness *like no one* for a human being; for this one. I am going to try, leaning over his shoulder while he was writing, to describe his strength. He is the witness of the witness; he lends the voice of all his experience, of all that he *knows*, to a witness who dies among us. "Each time unique, the end of the world" (Derrida).

Does *realizing* fail to penetrate the sheath of nothingness (Sartre) that encircles the solipsism of every-one, and that "run-for-your-life" of the "self," universal singular, whose first "testimony" as a survivor on a site of carnage is to shout at the cameras: "That could have been me! I thank God for sparing me"? The reality of the real is not "realizable," even when the real explodes ten meters from us at an airport. How can a writer make one realize, that is, pass the baton to witnesses of witnesses, when the *réalisateur* (director) today is the film- or video-maker, master of the "visualizable" reality of a real that has long since downgraded the *surreal* itself (and even in surrealist films)? Don't photos and recordings, zooms and enlargements, slow and fast motion, double and even quasi-subliminal mosaic-like exposures[8] disqualify scripturation?[9]

Unrealizability and the unrepresentable are left, face to face: can the former occur without the latter? Might it be the latter's fault if the former cannot succeed? Or, if there is not one thing that can escape presentation, being-in-the-presence-of — whether this be the divine in its burning bush or the "presence" of the world in the beauty of the poem (Bonnefoy) —, however "fleeting" the apparition may be (without any mystical "unsingable residue"),[10] the work again takes on the re-presentation of the "realizable," in "the sharing of the visible" achieved by a contemporary iconodulism, divided between the partisans of the visual image and those of language — or perhaps by their new alliance...

---

8   As for sexual bliss, at the other end of unrealizability, such and such film (I am referring to that supreme dud: *Malgré la nuit [Despite the Night]*) desperately insists on having the voyeur *glide* in everywhere; worms itself in as close as possible, *mutely* and intentionally as close as possible (thus technology-dependent), to mouths kissing and skins touching each other — even as it ideologically amplifies the moans of female pleasure.

9   The word "scripturation" translates the French neologism "écrituration," which emphasizes the materiality of the writing process and is based on the Portuguese term "escrituração," "writing" in the sense of "record," "recording." [TN]

10 Allusion to Paul Celan's poem "Singbarer Rest" ("Singable Remnant"). [TN]

In comes the performative: —

"To perform" would be synonymous with "to realize." Perhaps it is appropriate to hear the injunction in English first, whence performance comes to us, or rather comes back to us, surrounded by its lexical family (perform, performing…). The Anglo-American "performs" even more than the French "realizes." We know how great is the vogue (I almost said "discovery," or rediscovery)[11] that accompanies, amplifies, establishes, the regime of *performativity*, the influence and glory of Austin.

Yet where poetry is concerned, the performative formula switches the terms of the famous Austinian title (in its French iteration),[12] since poetry is *when doing is saying*.[13] The poem does (*poieï, poïema*, is its name); its doing is a saying. It says what a thing does when it does that which it is like. In the case of Ponge, for example, the oyster does the oyster, and the sun, the sun. The proper *doing* of the poem is its *techne*, its operation that says what a thing does by being like itself: love by making love,[14] for instance.

Poetry's other doing is its *prattein* (its praxis), of which I won't say anything here, when the poetic act (action, activity) tries to transform a circumstance into that which it can say; to act within the circumstance through a "reading" or in any other way. What remains to be analyzed is the conjunction (the re-union) of this *poieïn* and this *prattein*.

---

11 Since the invention, administration and practice of the sacraments ("*ex opere operato*") are as old as Christianity ("This is my body"), and since their "theological" study fills an immense library, more replete with in-octavos than that of *The Name of the Rose*, even if filming it would be less exciting…

12 Austin's *How To Do Things With Words* was translated into French (by Gilles Lane) as *Quand dire, c'est faire* (*When Saying Is Doing*). [TN]

13 As we know, "c'est quand" [literally: "it's when"] launches the puerile, childish definition (presentation) of the exemplary; as in "poetry, it's when…" *Wie wenn* according to the Hölderlinian *incipit*.

14 In 18th-century parlance, in Marivaux for example, "You made love to me, and frankly that made me happy" (Jacqueline in *The Surprise of Love*) signifies: "You are courting me by speaking of love to me," which already the sexual adolescent of the 21st century can no longer hear. In this case, the Pongian doing would get us to tackle "Mimesis" again — which I cannot elaborate on here.

"Who if I cried out [...]?"[15] Writing encloses language in silence: what is called interiority. This *mother*-tongue vociferated amongst ourselves, or from myself-to-myself, down to the *inaudible*, mouth-moving, imperceptibly uttered, self-addressed mumbling which gives to every solitary walker the appearance of a lunatic, how can we make it heard? Mouchard brings it near in *Entangled*. Traveling across space, infinite distance, the immense interval, it arrives at and through *reading*, which has been silent since Ambrose and yet deafens the secluded reader, the "addressee."

Doesn't this aporia duplicate that of the Hegelian "sense certainty," all the more blatant since *sensation*, the myth of a pre-logical experience, the cult of "unmediated living" by way of sonorous yet aphasic images, institutes — like a sedition, like a Great Day's vigil of the people — the suspicion and contempt of "language"; the desire to do without it?

You don't feel what I feel. I am suffering, I am dying three feet from you (here the pronouns can be swapped), and you feel nothing! Emotion and sensitivity are shattered by viewing... But "testimony," deprived of the visible (or as we prefer to say today, the visual), reported, related, narrated, does not transport (no meta-phorical transport suffices) pain nor actual bliss into "the other." Its reality would have to travel through the infinite silence where sensation has disappeared, and then be "realized" inside someone else... People asked themselves, for a whole generation, about the *silence* of the deported, more incredible still in those of Auschwitz... The *what's the use* of speaking about the "unsayable," since it will not be "realized" and thus not be believed, seems to have sealed their lips on the untestifiable... until today's insurrection of victims rising from the earth, as in Signorelli's fresco, for a resurrection preceding eternal silence...

Too late, perhaps, since "the world" has become concentrationary, exiling, expatriating its refugees by the millions; both genocidal *and* negationist? Against which Mouchard's written clamor tries "one last time" to seek another form of testimony, an other cry of silence, perhaps even *more* desperate... But is it possible today, when the *réalisateur* has become the filmmaker, master of the real?

---

15   Mouchard uses these words, the first words of Rilke's first *Duino Elegy*, as a title for his study of "œuvres-témoignages." See page XII of the Introduction. [TN]

Powerlessness in every respect, but first in making oneself heard, and by oneself?[16]

A writing is not a cry of pain. Yet it suffers and endures not being able to be that. "This is not a cry." Written tears are crocodile tears (assuming that the "real" crocodile never cries). And every true condolence letter contorts itself for not being able to cry (or make cry). This intimate and intrinsic contrariness (pugnacity of oppugnancies and repugnance) within testimony deepens its infirmity; its constitutive weakness is such that there will always be negationism — it's within us!? — like a kind of ventriloquism of denial, of denegation (or rejection, or contempt) of what I am *in the process* of reading or writing. The "Yes, that's how it is!" must always confront and surmount the "I can't believe it."

What remains of what took place? "Nothing will have taken place"…? Or perhaps, as I sometimes have it: "Nothing… *will* have taken place."[17] We call "trace" what subsists, meaning a material fragment that is still (always) present in the perception of the living. All is ruin, the poem says, and the ruin is a spiritual contour: memorizable, thinkable. Scraps of utterances — which were uttered — create a picture for a reader. The "rest" is this constant (uninterrupted) materiality, that which fell under the tact of contact. The *Noli me tangere* to Magdalene and the "put your hand into my wound" to Thomas reinforce one another. Pass the past on to me; quotations and things. Quotations consist in their materiality. Things are things. Witnesses are things.

The staging (on the page) of the powerless "if I cried out," of the witnesses' witness's testimony, is typographical.

Intensities, tones, timbres, voices, reliefs, asides, suspension of exclamation, music of gasps, of sideration… the list begun here is inexhaustible. To cut one's own speech off and then take it back; to go on, interrupt… to pass underneath, pass ahead, raise or lower one's tone, this calligram of possible voices, this *neumatics* of emissions, quotations, evocations, offers itself to reading, which is to say in every instance to the capacity of a reader.

---

16 Did Greek theater achieve this in the 5th century BC? Terror and Pity on all sides? But it no longer is, in our "cities," a matter of *catharsis*.

17 The two phrases in French are "Rien n'aura eu lieu" and "Rien… aura eu lieu"; in the second one, a standard element of negation is missing, which reifies "Rien," making nothing something, so to speak. [TN]

In the same way that the modern technique of double exposure allowed cinema, and then *screenization* — technologies endlessly chasing innovation in their "high definition" — to mime our shredded existence, the burning-hot-cockles game of perceptive planes, here writing undertakes to transpose the sonority in which we live surrounded by voices, by silences, the unheard and the ultrasonic, by "cries and whispers," the muffled and the deafening…

Perhaps the art *(technè)* here has more affinity with the hidden camera than with the *throw of the dice*… Writing has to follow.

I will close with an "impression": the words' obstinate bumping up against the right "justification" for me changes the white margin into a Wailing Wall struck with clenched fists… And so, to recast the enigma one last time, the *partitioning*, which plays such a decisive role in Mouchard's understanding of "who Khaled was," is also *represented* by this beseeched wall.

Michel Deguy

Introduction

CLAUDE MOUCHARD is a deeply stirring poet, who writes like no one else. I first met him in 1996, shortly after the publication of *Enchevêtrée (Entangled)*. An unassuming, self-effacing man, he is little known by English-speaking readers, though he has long served as associate editor-in-chief of *Po&sie*, one of France's leading poetry journals, and published many important critical writings as well as three beautiful collections of poems: *Ici* (1986), *Perdre* (1979; 1989), *L'Air* (1997); the "pamphlet-poem" *Papiers!* (2007); and several series of poetic *Notes* (in *Po&sie* and elsewhere), selections from which are included in this book. Over the last ten years Mouchard's poems have remained as focused on what has been happening in the world as attuned to his inner experience, dealing largely with the plight of the exiled and homeless — an urgent problem of global consequence, as terrible events linked to the migrant crisis keep reminding us daily. Yet the quiet, ongoing *notation* of what Mouchard has come to call "political sensations," though always fed by and receptive of current information, has nothing to do with what is simply "new" or "passing." Rather, the radically innovative poetry that he offers, which began to appear as a kind of lyrical extension of (or supplement to) his last critical opus, *Qui si je criais…?*, a reflection on testimonial writings around 20th-century political catastrophes, is quite literally the work of a lifetime. It is an *œuvre-témoignage* in its own right, in which the poet refuses to advance his own voice alone, choosing rather to have it always accompany or let itself be shot through with the voices of others who have been or risk being silenced.

Upon encountering a highly singular poet whose paradoxical starting point is to refuse singularity, readers will perhaps not be surprised to learn that Mouchard has also worked for decades as a translator of other contemporary poets from several languages and many distant parts of the world (Japan and Korea in particular) — often in collaboration with the poets themselves or with other native speakers.[1] His current primary project has been to shepherd

---

[1] Thus, although Mouchard is only beginning to receive the recognition his work warrants in the West, he is quite well-known elsewhere — a book of his translated work was published in 2015 in China, and another will soon appear in Korea. *Qui si je criais…? Œuvres-témoignages dans les tourmentes du XXe siècle* (Laurence Teper, 2007) was translated into Chinese by Li Jinjia (*Shui, zai wo huhan shi… ershi shiji de jianzheng wenxue*. Shanghai: Presses Universitaires de l'Université Normale Supérieure de Huadong, 2015).

the translation and publication in *Po&sie* of poets from all over the African continent.² My aim in the following remarks will be to elucidate some of the strong yet intricate ties linking Mouchard's life as a politically engaged critic and translator with his profoundly original poetry.

How is Mouchard's poetic writing linked to his practice of translation? *Entangled*,³ the opening work in this volume, though more intimate and less concerned with "others" and "the world" than the subsequent *Papers!* or *Notes*, already shows this link very well. For it manages to mark and make us feel the loss of an other's identity through language, across a widening divide. *Entangled* brings alive and sets in a complex form the ephemeral circumstances, thoughts, and feelings surrounding the final words uttered by the poet's mother, who lost her ability to speak due to Alzheimer's. The poem thus exposes not only the high stakes but also the stumbling blocks inherent in all translation, in that it lays bare the difficulty and range of experiences a writer can have in trying to seize, interpret, and transform another person's words into a different mode of expression — another way of thinking and speaking — and emphasizes at the same time how much our experience of things is mixed with that of a given language form.

In the fall of 2003, I asked Mouchard to tell me about the context surrounding the creation of this poem. He answered that what he was trying to achieve was a "*déroulement*," an "unwinding" of the elements of reality embedded in (and thus "entangled" with) those particular sentences that his mother last spoke in attempting to articulate something about her dog — compelling yet hard-to-grasp words, which he had often been tempted to recount and which had remained seared in his memory.

> What am I trying to do with such sentences?
> "Realize" is the expression that comes to me. The lasting hope, which makes me write around them and for them, is that of realizing. Might it be in the sense that we tend to say, when witnessing certain events or hearing certain words, that we do

---

2   See the two volumes of this ambitious enterprise, *Afriques 1*, *Po&sie*, Nºs 153–154 (Paris: Belin, 2016), and *Afriques 2*, *Po&sie*, Nºs 157–158 (Paris: Belin, 2017).
3   *Enchevêtrée*, published in the journal *Le Nouveau Commerce* (Paris), Cahier 100 (Automne – Hiver 1996) 47–67.

not "realize" or had not "realized" in the moment, that time is needed to "realize" what has been seen or heard?

In one sense, Mouchard's aim to consciously seize, recapture, reconstitute a subjective reality that has been lost in time seems close to the project articulated in Proust's *Le Temps retrouvé*, in the famous lines where the narrator presents all great writing as a kind of translation:

> [...] the only true book, a great writer does not have, in the usual sense, to invent it, since it exists already in each one of us, but to translate it. The duty and the task of the writer are those of the translator.[4]

But there is also something fundamentally *dialogical* in Mouchard's way of writing and reconstituting reality through language. His texts manifest, I would say, an unsettled *performative* approach, and yet one that also underlines — and this is what is perhaps most unusual — the value and necessity of *communication* in every sense of the term.

Thus, in *Entangled*, the unwinding of words seeks not only to preserve fragments of self-expression, be they the mother's or the poet's own, but also to represent the necessarily *open-ended* exchange that takes place as one tries to move (in) language between disparate voices, different ways of speaking. Rather than seizing a certain, definitive reality within a fixed and sealed monument, Mouchard's writing seeks to set itself in motion and remain open through time. This ambitious project, immediately felt as one reads through the poems of this collection, was formulated quite precisely in Mouchard's letter on *Enchevêtrée*:

> But the words quoted are precisely the ones I don't need to realize. If they stay in my memory, it is by radiating — wounding, irresorbable — an excess of reality.
>
> It's rather all of the rest of language and thought that seems to me affected by a lack of reality. And it is in relation

---

[4] Marcel Proust, *A la recherche du temps perdu*, ed. Jean-Yves Tadié, *Œuvres complètes IV* (Paris: Gallimard, 1989) 469. Unless otherwise noted, French quotes in this volume are rendered in English by the translator.

to those words — cited as inclusions — that I try to realize, to create sentences that realize, and realize themselves. Or rather it is a whole volume that should then, around these quoted words, take form, and hold — fragile, but real. This volume should be made of sentences that move in relation to one another, balance each other and suspend each other reciprocally.

Some actually should be whispered, hardly audible, others should be felt in one blow — yes, like a vibrating blow —, even while remaining obstinately, as sentences, unfoldable (so as to deliver, if one wishes, a whole content).

And this volume, finally, would not be exactly closed. At least it should leave the impression that other sentences could still come there to play with those that are written and printed.

Indeed, as is obvious at first glance, the complex typographical play of *Entangled* — its varied use of lines and spaces, of capitals and of roman and italic type — *makes visible* and ideally, in performance, also *audible* the inextricable interrelations of a musical, multidimensional reality that is at the same time very abstract and very concrete. In this respect, and in the general complexity of its form, the poem recalls Mallarmé's *Un coup de dés*.

In *Entangled*, however, the subject matter is deeply personal, and the mode far from hypothetical: the roman type generally recounts the basic true "story" of the poet's mother's last utterance, whereas the italics convey a rush of afterthoughts or a running gloss on that story, elements that the poet fills in as a response to thinking about it. Sometimes the italicized remarks take on the form of meta-linguistic questioning, of analytic commentary, while at other times they supplement and develop concrete details in the narrative. But there are also several instances where the roles of the roman type and the italics appear crossed, representing, perhaps, the inevitable *entanglement* of the different kinds of reflection — on experienced fact, but also on language and representation — that are at work in the poem and occurring at many different levels.

Mouchard's poem is monolingual, yet it unmasks what any process of translation actually requires but ultimately hides: a constant shuttling not just between different languages, but between speakers, voices, ways of speaking. Its dialogical character inevitably produces a hybrid poetic genre, a cross between a reflexive narrative, a dramatic staging, and a lyrical and meditative evocation. As such, *Entangled* also fulfills its performative function, offering a "requiem," a musical rite honoring the poet's mother's memory upon her death. The poet releases his mother's memory along with his own by purifying it, by fully recognizing first its loss and then allowing all that lingers from her voice in a whispered chant to return to the light and air. And, in a paradoxical development that is wholly natural yet surprising, this intimate preservation of the mother's words, this honoring of the mother's life that leads to a new form of writing, ultimately also gives rise in Mouchard's works to a wider, though still private, still protected space that preserves and embraces other lives, other voices within the poet's community, reaching, through conversation, a dramatic opening of poetry to the world.

* * *

We begin to see this paradoxically intimate socio-political dimension of Mouchard's dynamic poetics quite clearly in his pamphlet-poem *Papers!*[5] This work, published in 2007, expands the dialogical character of *Entangled* and announces the open-ended polyphony of the vast series of *Notes*, which manage to integrate a deeply rooted lyric within a new and relentless form of analysis, a questioning of all orders of relations within the self and between the self and others. Presenting itself explicitly as a tract and published in tandem with Mouchard's last critical masterwork (*Qui si je criais…*), *Papers!* at first appears less grounded in the poet's ongoing life story than *Entangled*, or the *Notes* that follow. *Papers!* is in some ways a more polemical and self-contained work, insofar as it remains anchored in a very specific political crisis — the beginning of the influx of and hardening against people seeking asylum in Europe —;

---

5   *Papiers! pamphlet-poème* (Paris: Editions Laurence Teper, 2007); an earlier version of this text also appeared in *Po&sie*, N⁰ 117–118 (Paris: Éditions Belin, 2006). For an acute and far-reaching critical analysis of this poem and its relation to "*Qui si je criais*" and Mouchard's other works, see Martin Rueff's essay, "« A l'ici, même lointain, la poésie touche seule » — Sur Claude Mouchard, *Qui si je criais? Œuvres-témoignages dans les tourmentes du XXᵉ siècle et Papiers!*," in *Agenda de la pensée contemporaine*, N⁰s 9–10 (winter 2007; spring 2008).

and also presents itself to "us," even as it questions who "we" are, as a call, a cry even, for action.

Opening with summaries and quotations of all-too-fleeting October 2006 news reports on the arrival in Europe of refugees from the slaughter in Darfur despite strenuous efforts by the European community to keep them out, the poem fixes our attention in an increasingly personal way on the miserable conditions of illegal immigrants and other homeless people in contemporary France. What does it mean to expel, to ignore, the "others" who inhabit our space, those who live among us within the boundaries of our countries, our cities, our lives? When we pretend not to even see them, and thus refuse to acknowledge their humanity, no less welcome them, what does this do to us?

In *Papers!* Mouchard simultaneously registers what is reported, what is happening around him, and the effects he observes, on himself and others, of tightening borders, the difficulty of obtaining shelter, and the egregious conditions of those who remain homeless in his country. He thus ultimately reflects as much on what it means to have as not to have identity *papers*. Necessary and life-defining as they can be, these documents ultimately say nothing about who we are. Yet, contrary to what one might expect, poetry is not at all for Mouchard a vehicle for "identity" politics. "Nothing," he stated in a recent interview about his work in *Mediapart*, a French online news organization, "is, perhaps, so anti-identitary as poetry and the translation of poetry."[6] And the paradoxical tension inherent for him in composing a political poem — the text is political because it clearly points to a problem within the public space and moves us to wish to resolve it, but remains poetic insofar as it does not pretend to resolve the problem in this way — becomes especially trenchant in the last pages of *Papers!* For the poet's most moving and striking encounter is with a mysterious "frozen man," clearly of African origin, yet who may or may not have papers, and whom the poet ardently wishes to help, but feels he cannot begin to know. The motif of the poet's ever-accumulating debt to those he reaches out to is brought to a climax in this part of the poem.

---

6 Claude Mouchard: "Par le poème, il y a des événements qui ne cessent plus d'arriver." Interview with Patrice Beray, August 11, 2014 (www.mediapart.fr/print/438793).

The "pamphlet-poem" literally closes as the poet realizes that his drawing attention to the problem of political outcasts in an outcry is not simply a rhetorical positioning or a manner of poetic writing; it converges also (as through a "demon of analogy") with an actual incident of his crying out, though it felt like a dream; a shouting at the border, which might not only have been vain, but have had a negative effect. This involuntary cry broke out when, returning from a visit to China, the poet saw a fellow passenger — who had sat next to him during the long journey and whom he had tried to befriend — hassled at the airport and detained, not because he was without papers, but because he had inadequate ones. Conscious that the most powerful gesture a writer can make is to move and place us in front of a problem whether or not he can resolve it, Mouchard highlights at the end of *Papers!* the all-pervasive quandary that is the subject of this poem — the crisis these documents symbolize and entail both within and outside every country and every city, endlessly raising questions for us all.

In this final movement of the poem we again see the crucial role of typography in Mouchard's musical-political poetic; for the details of the event unfold in an especially complex pattern, combining the effects of not only verse and prose and several different type sizes of roman and italic print, but also a passage of verse justified on the right, where the voice seems actually to come from a different place, to be situated elsewhere, as it conveys his efforts at "*fraternisation*" with his traveling companion, including breaking bread with him on the plane. Sewn through this ending, we also find underscored in boldface a rather clear, if reflexive, statement, a primary motif, which conveys what the poet has been trying to grapple with throughout the poem. The boldface begins by positing a question among various lines and styles of type:

LIKE A KNOCK ON (or a **grip on**) **THE SHOULDER**

what took hold of me?

and similarly sews through the last lines of the poem the following suspended response:

INTRODUCTION

> **This was [...]**
>
> **not [...] a matter of no papers,**
> **but rather one of insufficient papers ... [?],**
>
> [...] *it was then* [...]
>
> *crying out for real* — [...]
>
>   **Nothing,** [...]
>
>   nor
>
> **the question:**
>   [...] **nothing stops — there**

This answer, which refuses to close the question (even as it gathers a complex narrative that unwinds all around it), asserts as much about the edges or boundaries of the poem — its simultaneous need for and rejection of drawing strong lines — as it does about the political "papers" to which it also refers. Correspondences between life and its representation in writing must somehow be realized partially and provisionally, even if any grasp of the whole of them will by definition be unthinkable, just as political problems are irresolvable once and for all. They demand our ongoing attention even as they divide it, just as borders and boundaries separate "we" who supposedly belong within certain places from others who are invariably, inextricably in there with "us" too.

    The political dimension of this poem, its action, which dares to assert itself and bind itself to a certain moment in time, and yet does so in a way that proves somehow enduring, announces the creation of a new open-ended *œuvre-témoignage*, which Mouchard has been pursuing for many years already, and will continue to pursue as long as he lives.

                          *   *   *

    This new form of literary testimonial is the prodigious assemblage of *Notes* that Mouchard has begun publishing with increasing frequency, in multiple venues in response to readers' demands, over the last several years. The first series presented here, "*From Darfur to the Loire with Ousmane to begin*" originally appeared in *Po&sie* in 2008, while the second, entitled "*& whether this is living?*," was first published in 2010 in *Le Grand Huit*, a collection honoring the 80th birthday of Michel Deguy (the author of this volume's preface).[7] That Mouchard chose those contexts among others in which to present this extraordinary ongoing work makes sense insofar as Deguy and he have long been collaborators (through their editorial partnership in *Po&sie*) in the effort to open up French poetry to a multitude of voices. A primary and unusual feature of Mouchard's poetic *Notes* is that they freely give voice not only to others whom the poet encounters, but also to a wealth of literary and paraliterary texts. The title, "*& whether this is living*," is in fact a quote from Virginia Woolf's diary; and within the body of that text, as in other fragments of the *Notes*, we often come across not only words spoken in conversation and media snippets, but short and long quotations from an astonishing array of works of world literature, sometimes with poetic glosses, sometimes without, but always illuminated by prismatic reflections linking them with the poet's words and each other.

This infinite, open-ended dialogue, which the *Notes* capture in a deliberately partial way — Mouchard insists they should not be published as a whole and presents them *serially*, with occasional reprisals and reworkings of certain passages to prevent their mutation into a definitive "work" —,[8] reflects the poet's deep concern with the central fact and dynamic of relations in human life, not only relations among people and texts, languages, and cultures, but also relations between various states *within* the subject and thus the poetic "self." The "other" within (like the other without) is not only shown, but warmly welcomed, given a home in Mouchard's poetry, and this corresponds to a fundamental feature of the man, which Deguy pointedly evokes in "Penser-à," a piece devoted to Mouchard that winds up *L'Amour de l'Air*, a collection honoring the poet.

---

7   See *Po&sie*, № 125 (Belin, 2008) 113–123; *Le Grand Huit* (Le Bleu du ciel, 2010) 149–155; also the journal *Fario* (2010: № 8, 53–108; 9, 223–273); the website *Poezibao* (March–April & November 2012); *Po&sie*, № 152 (2015), 10–28. One finds antecedents of the *Notes* in other publications as well, for example, in the last few pages of Mouchard's poetry collection *L'Air* (Belval: Circé, 1997), or in "*Dans quoi?*" (*Po&sie*, № 105, 2003, 63–75).

8   See, for example, in the *Notes*, the deliberate reinsertion of a passage from the first series (pages 59–60) toward the opening of the last one (pages 107–108).

For Deguy, Mouchard emblematizes what "thinking of" entails both in its subjective and objective dimensions. As poet, as critic, as translator, he helps us to realize that to think of something is generally also to think of someone and vice-versa:

> To Claude Mouchard, I would like to offer (dedicate? propose?) some thoughts, some reflections. Which ones? Why?
> Often one thinks of someone at the same time that one thinks (of) something; or one thinks "things," and almost simultaneously one thinks of someone, to whom they belong. "Association of ideas." Thought turns toward a recipient, who might have inspired it. The donee is the donor. I often think of Claude in thinking of things I am going to say.[9]

What does Deguy think of when writing about Mouchard? Of the need for real "*dia-logue*," multiple interlocutors moving together, as opposed to against one another, to replace conventional polemics; and of the necessity for true exchange, "*travail comme-un*" (common work or work as-one), to move through trouble and create *rapprochement*; of Mouchard's authentic *résistance* to political and social evils; and of his friendship, his abiding closeness as a former colleague and co-editor of *Po&sie*; but above all of his particular way of writing, as a "weaver of intertexts," a "testifier to testimonials"; and of the depth and breadth of his commitment to translation.

> Translation is his favorite gesture perhaps. Because it is of the order of hospitality. It welcomes, it is strangely indebted: the debt of the translator accumulates! He settles it by incurring it.[10]

---

9 Michel Deguy, "Penser-à," in *L'Amour de l'air. Pour Claude Mouchard* (Paris: Scripta, 2002) 35.
10 "Penser-à," 44.

We know that welcoming the strange, the foreign, within one's own language can indeed be an ideal of literary translation.[11] This is part of what distinguishes it from utilitarian, flattening translation, since the very function of language and writing is not to wipe out difference, but to delight in it and form bridges between languages, and between people. Here is how Deguy puts this, in concluding his remarks on Mouchard:

> Language is what passes through, and allows passage; it's the bridge over the abyss; the *inter*.
>
> To speak of the "*un*translatable" is to refer to the heterogeneity of "cultures," of *ethnicities* [...]. Does not thus refer so much to languages, which are on the contrary essentially passing from one to the next, in *trans*, made to speak among themselves, to "translate" one another.
>
> Language is that through which cultures in trans-action pass the most easily; easy, negotiable difference, allowing passages, which have always been used, for the "communication" of vessels; whereas what does not pass through at all, or less so, what hesitates or is loath to pass through, it's the "proper," taste, history, intimate conviction, the "god." Cannot pass, except by way of inter-locution in trans-lation; speaking-to-each-other by learning the language of others.[12]

As the *Notes* dramatically illustrate, what generally applies to language and translation defines all the more keenly the poet in Mouchard's case, acting like a radical imperative as much within his own lyrical self-expression as in his manner of dealing with others and the world. Everywhere the poet's hospitality is indeed conceived in terms of a debt. So that even "*& whether this is living?*," the second *Notes* series here, which drifts far away from the focus of the first one, *begins again* with the words of "Ousmane," pseudonym of the refugee

---

11   See for example, A. Berman, *La Traduction et la lettre ou l'auberge du lointain* (Paris: Seuil, 1999) 75.
12   Michel Deguy, "Penser-à," 49.

from Darfur whom we come to know in "*From Darfur to the Loire*," and whom Claude and Hélène Mouchard actually hosted for eight years in their home; and in this second instance we find Ousmane once more insisting, in precise, if broken, French, that the life he is still experiencing in exile (alongside the poet and living in his house) is not his own:

"**no**," says Ousmane: "**this not-my-a-life.**"

This striking feature of Mouchard's *Notes*, which conceive of poetry as hospitality and as an ongoing debt to the lives and voices of others, appears all the more crucial when we recognize that their publication, or their emergence as creative works *for others*, so closely accompanied the poet's concrete day-to-day efforts to help Ousmane retrieve a life, a worldly effort that was successful to an important degree and also implied a poetic process and commitment of Mouchard's *whole person* to explore and capture, in the moment, what this refugee's life with his own and that of others has been. This trajectory is suggested as much by the first two series of *Notes* presented here as by others not included in this volume, such as "*Avec la peau d'une autre vie*" ("With the skin of another life," published by the French poetry website *Poezibao* in November of 2012), where the reader learns the latest news about Ousmane, discovers that a series of "miracles" (Ousmane's word) enabled him to reunite with his family in the Sudan and to buy them a house in Khartoum. In the final passages of that text, we are also brought into the poet's inquiry as to how and why his new work seems destined to present itself serially and in installments, in the manner of the *feuilleton* narrative genre.

"With Ousmane": a series?
Since his arrival here — July 2007 — "at home," even his story has been a series which day after day I will have tried to follow with "notes."
These notes have been enmeshed with what has happened, and doesn't stop happening…
Heterogeneous and jumpy — under the impact of various and unexpected news.
Enmeshed with decisions that life with O. has demanded.

> Or "localizing": insisting day after day on recreating and cautiously testing the "here-and-now."
> Or the "with" or the "between."
> Attacking what churlish substance of dirty ice?[13]

If the internal and outer structure of the *Notes* can't be wholly fixed, so as to retain their openness to the contingencies of life, the structure of the serial fragments must be set at the moment of publication in order to fulfill another aspect of their function, which is to welcome new readers and embrace them in the dynamic of a work-ever-in-progress. The original, open-ended movement must be somehow preserved even as its parts are revisited and presented in print; lines must be drawn and redrawn in the sand, somehow conveying their own potential for displacement so as to ensure that they will be *taken up again* by the poet himself, as well as his readers.

Tragically, the "here-and-now" presented in "*Tout seul, Khaled?*," the final *Notes* series in this book, is that the Darfuri refugee, who lived with Mouchard for several years and whom readers come to know so intimately in the *Notes* as "Ousmane," died of a sudden heart attack in the Spring of 2015 in Mouchard's house, so that the poet became suddenly faced with entangling this cherished young man's last words (as he previously had the last utterances of his mother) with his own, and with wondering whether and how he would be able to continue his life's work. Certainly he has, though the poetry he now writes reaches out in new directions, to embrace the words and artworks of others who risk being silenced. Time then clearly marks but does not change the fundamental nature of Mouchard's notes. And the only crucial transformation that occurs through the *Notes* series represented here is that following his friend's death, Mouchard no longer feels obliged to shield his identity with a fictional name (which, the first series told us, the refugee had requested and chosen); so that in the last series he finally emerges as himself, Khaled — the true interlocutor of the poet, now fully vested with the truth and value of the poetic exchange.

---

13   « *Avec la peau d'une autre vie* » [*Feuilleton*], in *Poezibao* (November 12–December 7, 2012) (http://poezibao.typepad.com/files/claude-mouchard-avec-la-peau-dune-autre-vie-notes-poezibao-2012.pdf).

Thus, no matter where we turn in the *Notes*, we see that a dialogical baring of the self's and others' responses to the demands of human life, yet one still striving to embrace all of its dimensions — becomes at once the aim and method of Mouchard's poetic work, a reality-ideal, which at the same time must and can never be achieved. All the *Notes* fragments speak of the relation-forming and deforming network that is life, be this through the recurrent motifs of the poet's "live" exchanges with Ousmane/Khaled; through his final conversation with his slowly expiring mother; or through literary exchanges with statements from other writers and readers — as we saw in the quotation from Woolf's diary, which concludes with her commitment to read Proust, or as we see in a partially quoted poem by Ritsos, where Mouchard's gloss tentatively asks whether the image of a man cut-off from speaking in a camp does not implicate the final and most basic severance:

> "**something white, infinitely white**": color of terror? of the
> death of all connection, of the most elementary trust?

We thus get the overarching sense from Mouchard's work that life holds us as much as we hold it by means of spoken, written, and gestural *communication lines* tying us to the presence of others, who inhabit us within and without; others who wait for us; hence the still primordial role of mothers, who insist that life, being something which they give, must also be somehow preserved and returned to them.

As Vincent Pélissier, editor of a 2010 series entitled *La vie douce et la terreur* in the art journal *Fario*, remarks: if Mouchard chooses to publish his *Notes* in this unconventionally open-ended way, it is because he refuses to settle or limit the questions that concern him: "an innumerable crowd of beings and of books, of poems, of testimonies enters here without rest, without respite, assailing the present, not to establish it, but rather to trouble it." The poet seeks to keep all he writes, all he writes about, burning within himself and his readers, as this particular series' title also suggests by emphasizing a fundamental polarity in all human experience: the tender familiarity of the everyday in "la vie douce," (the good life) and the moments of catastrophe, political and personal, of fear and horror, "la terreur," which simultaneously interrupt ordinary life and make it all the more precious. This is a paradox everywhere evoked in Mouchard's poems.

There is no sewing up, no neat packaging so that the reader can come away with a comforting sense of how this essential conflict can be resolved.

The *Notes* are thus unsettling in every aspect of their presentation; as Pélissier aptly comments, though they may recall certain qualities of the journal, sketchbook, or essay, they do not fit easily into any of these writing genres, appearing rather as a

> sum in perpetual reshuffling under the effect of pushes or forces, of ruptures, but also of deposits, of accumulations, of alluviums of readings or encounters, eroded by time and by reworking [...].
>
> A continual and active interrogation on the violence implied in the "making of a work" ensures for this text a kind of horizontality without edges, deprives it of whatever might be linked to an architecture or a plan. No overhang would a priori allow one to envision, surmount, or overdetermine these notes and the questions that cross through and cleave them.

No doubt, it is this radical refusal of a whole and settled form, and this blending of the hard and soft, of terror with intimate sweetness, that create such a profound opening within the *Notes*' readers, an effect which Pélissier (a prominent Parisian psychiatrist) also pointedly describes:

> I remember the shock that was triggered by the encounter with these texts [...]. In reading them, I felt myself suddenly cut off, isolated from the familiar world in which were passing, in the heat of August, ordinary and simple days. Few books produce such upheavals.[14]

By allowing us access to a life work ever in progress, but open to interruption and turmoil, Mouchard forces fundamental ruptures in our reading habits,

---

14   Vincent Pélissier, remarks following the publication of the *Notes* series *La vie douce et la terreur* in *Fario*, Nº 8 (spring 2010) 109–110.

and, first of all, in our tendency to categorize and compartmentalize disparate voices within different kinds of reading and empirical experiences. This process of simultaneously exposing and bringing down the walls that typically structure and divide life and literary writing is what makes Mouchard's poetry so original and so moving. And its trajectory (as the poet himself notes) follows the arc of his life in a manner that is at once organic:

> Mine, the gift of age: **the internal walls of flesh brown invisible in the heart** are crumbling.
> To realize, in words like these, the thawing of old interior partitions: here it is, at last, the sudden, unexpected pink tide sizzling with possibilizations…,
> fecundity *in extremis*.

and the very opposite of completely natural — self-conscious, reflective, and deliberative:

> Belatedly, I recognized that I was "partitioning" between, on one side, what was happening successively with people (over years, decades) who found shelter here and, on the other side, my "literary" endeavors. Did I need to? Was I afraid that "poetic" writing would become the target of imperatives — be they — especially — "generous" ones — that it might accept to become, in this sense, predictable… And yet, today, I am knocking down those walls…[15]

Paradoxically, this inner collapse of compartmentalization also leads Mouchard and his readers to a new experience of time that embraces rather than eschews circularity, as we see in the following passage from a later series also printed in *Fario*, entitled *L'ordinaire* (which both includes and extends the end of *"& whether this is living?"*), where the poet emphasizes how time seems at once to be catching up with and slowing itself down for him, adapting to

---

15 « *Avec la peau d'une autre vie* », in *Poezibao* (November 2012), mouchard-avec-la-peau-dune-autre-vie-notes-poezibao (downloaded file, 15 and 23–24).

his life by almost, but not quite, breaking, in a polar relation to its forward-driving movement during childhood, where the road seemed to leap up to greet the wheel of his speeding bike.

> **Time now, was beginning to tenderly extend out of itself —**
> not forward, but there, beneath... the very advance of existence, realizing this advance itself by curbing it, by slowing it down almost to the point of stopping it...
>
> like *a road of time gone by in childish exaltation, at dusk, running along the Loire, the asphalt unfolding*
> *elastic orange called up-snatched under the tire while the glow of the frontlight attached to the fender jumped*
> *revealing itself no less elastic than the tire*
>
> time, stretching itself in place by becoming indefinitely cracked, grey-whitened, without breaking...[16]

In this passage, as with the image of the child on the bike just taking off (under the warning cries of his mother) at the end of "*& whether this is living?*," the italics marking speed are framed within the more staid movement of the roman type. What is more, the entire note fragment takes form "underneath" the bold-face type that signals the circular extension of time as the text's primary motif. In this way, the whole passage recreates for the reader a kind of score and musical dynamic that encourages also our circulation within the *durée* of the text.

Typography and placement thus play a crucial role in the paradox of setting Mouchard's *Notes* as a work-in-progress, as a poem that presents itself as open to performance and to chance. For it is the typographical composition and layout that impose order and hierarchy to these lines, even as they suggest that they might have already or may still come together in a different order elsewhere. The boldface type obviously provides the clearest statement throughout

---

16   *L'ordinaire*, in *Fario*, Nº 9 (2010) 227.

the various series of *Notes*, offering a kind of spine around which the roman type turns, while the italics offer a third register of spatial and temporal hierarchy, tangibly conjoining the thought process with that of musicalisation, the poetic transformation of words into music.

And the politics surging from these *Notes*? I have tried to show that by fully welcoming others and Khaled in particular — a stranger who became a friend and an anchor for his writing, through a long and careful process undertaken by both men to establish an intimate, familial relationship without ceasing to recognize cultural differences — Mouchard's work offers a new and inspiring model for engagement.

How to begin? No formula is suggested in the pages gathered here. Each reader is left to respond to these unusual texts from the depth of his or her own impressions, as Deguy's preface so beautifully does, leaving us with the image of Mouchard's right justification as a kind of wailing wall. And yet, how to begin? is perhaps the first necessary question, the one that Mouchard relentlessly asks himself even as he advances, drawing for us the picture of a changing world: a world where solitude and private space remain crucial to artistic expression, but which also demands intimate and far-reaching communication with others. Global culture has evolved so that identity is always "imbricated." Mouchard's poems allow us to hear and be moved by some of the voices that interrupt our own even as they risk not being heard; and through ruptures, interstices, and textual spaces that transpose real political and social differences, they bear witness to everything that imposes yet still emerges from silence.

Acknowledgements

The translator wishes to thank Claude Mouchard, Rainer J. Hanshe, Alessandro Segalini, Richard Sieburth, and Jonathan Baillehache for their generous help with various parts and aspects of this work; and, especially, François Cornilliat for his careful reading and countless suggestions, which immeasurably improved the whole.

The texts assembled in this volume were reproduced and translated from the following original publications:

- *Enchevêtrée*. *Le Nouveau Commerce* (Paris), № 100 (Automne – Hiver 1996) 47–67.
- *Papiers! pamphlet-poème* (Paris: Éditions Laurence Teper, 2007).
- "Du Darfour à la Loire avec Ousmane pour commencer." *Po&sie*, № 125 (Paris: Belin, 2008) 113–123.
- "« & si c'est cela vivre ? »." *Le Grand Huit. Pour fêter les 80 ans de Michel Deguy* (Coutras: Le Bleu du ciel, 2010) 149–155.
- "Aube perpétuelle ?" Title created for the purpose of the present publication. Text first published in *Poezibao* (http://poezibao.typepad.com/poezibao) as installments 4 through 8 of the feuilleton "« Et si c'était cela vivre ? »" (April 2–11, 2012).
- "Tout seul, Khaled ?" *Po&sie*, № 152 (Paris: Belin, 2015) 10–28.

Entangled

SHE STUMBLES. Her lower lip droops.
It's the old distrust flaring up again, but with a doubt, I think, completely new.
Flecks of ash are floating, under the beams, the enormous roof.

———————————————————————————

Weave a story out of these instants? I wanted to (conversations ...)
just afterwards — but cut myself off right away.

———————————————————————————

Her doubt dazzles. "YOU ...," she says,
standing in the room's doorway.
She extends her right index finger, thin, trembling ...

Metallic gray hair twisting in the light, rough, coarse —
each strand could be counted.
Would she want to stay frozen?

Behind her the next room is, almost horizontally, lit. Flowing in, through the bay-window, the sun of an early March evening — spread out pale and cold on the fields where last year's stubble lingers, the dried remains of corn stalks.

———————————————————————————

Does she, from this point on, feel the air any differently? What does she see, in each minute, fibrillating or granulating? Will space stop being navigable for her?

The present, written here: crude.
It tries, short-winded, to hook these sentences (the time they take) on ... or in ... what happened then

(or in what should not be allowed, merely, to have happened — at least not if what she attempted, thus IN EXTREMIS, *must not remain blocked there.)*

The radio, barely audible in one of the bedrooms. Door half-opened; draft.

Coming (say): across the likely foggy hollow formed by the nearby fields, a call — of cow, or chicken — or, from yet further off, carried by bursts of wind, the minuscule and incessant snippings of hundreds of guinea-fowl under corrugated roofs.

She holds her hands clasped at the height of her chest,
a silhouette where other silhouettes are dancing.

She depends entirely now, distrustful, exposed, on a gesture that I will make;
take her by the elbow,
guide her slowly to the stained red armchair in front of the newly built brick fireplace.

Is it doubt that breathes through her

or, very old, a desire to believe that
    is trying to re-kindle
        — in order to pass beyond, vanish in a glow of embers…

Clearly, there is nothing familiar to her anymore. Everything turns around on her, against her, stops her.

Everything coarsens
      (grayish? or wildly colored? *Neither I nor she have access to what she feels*)

and sticks to her face,
        slithers on her watering corneas.

At least, in this too vast and too temporary room
        (a stable's naked frame:
        soft masses of dust hanging on splinters of wood
        continuously undo themselves,
        white throbs in the air)

where I was wrong to take her and where I must now guide her gently, there is one thing that she discovers with joy:
the fire.
Suddenly she speaks of it, in a barely audible voice.

Noise in the fireplace:
burnt wood collapsing or metal creaking as it dilates.

Flames — whose surges she begins to comment on (with small, crumb-like, exalted, almost imperceptible exclamations)
        as (wind rushing in) they suddenly
        illuminate her, heat her —
she,
    sitting as she is now,
would never tire of them
    (does she sense at the same time that which, obscure, avid,
        has already insinuated itself
        and envelops and confuses her thoughts?)

———————————————————————

But all of a sudden, what she notices even more keenly, it's —
      back from the fields and the hedges (bushes without leaves, long
      flattened grasses yellowed by winter, crawling mint stems,
      and the tracks of field mice or grass snakes) —

her black dog
which, short and tail awag, nudges her hand with her snout.

"DOG"? That's saying too much.
For precisely, as her mumblings, now garrulous, bump into one another,
she does not use this name.

Could it be that she no longer has access to this word? It seems rather *(was I sure of it then?)*
that she *(was avoiding it)*
AVOIDS IT.

───────────────

THIS SMALL, DARK, WARM BODY, jumpy, prancing,
gleaming with an ugly *(for me?)* dampness

belongs obviously to the more-than-known, to the "made for,"
        to all that which, *suburban houses and yards,*
        well-traced streets,
        raspberry and rose-bushes, pyracanthas,
        believes itself to be absolutely predictable,
        would like to see itself *(rough-cast edges, dull lines)*
        shot through with obviousness,
but springs from it, there,
        uttered … in the barn (the void) by this old mouth,

        uttering in order to
        flash-realize the banality
        flesh formed in the air only,
        by her gasps and gestures,

        and eats — through its power for mixing and simplification —
        the name I still might want to give it …

...fluctuation,
(burning saliva)...
would all words be at that moment
potentially affected, softly weakened?

Hasn't she, in what she will never name again,
   ...I feel it less while looking at
   the dog
   (even though, snuggled up against her,
   she is the precise result of what she wanted)

   than while trying, from the brief hints
   of her whispers, her formless gestures

   to discern or to condense
   (along with her, but differently)
   right in front of her face or very close to her hands
   in the bluish evening

   a stain, unstable

slipped in and kept (dissimulated?) for years,
a remnant of her oldest
   (contracted, over there, during the first world war)

ANIMAL

ALLIANCES OR REPULSIONS

— those which, inherited, age-old,

risked — in what a life like hers had become, not being able to go any further

and having to remain
unchanged and cruelly starving,
in the depths of her childhood — where very slow time emerged,

where childish-animal odors and breaths would lie forever in wait,

    contacts
        flank against flank or thigh,
           skin or little girl's skirt
                against wool and short coat
                    in the twilight, sheep and dogs

            brought together on the steep edge of the plateau
                and, emanating from the frozen boulder crashes
            opened just before night

        (I had, as a child, felt it in her long before
                knowing what it was),

    terror — iron teeth.

———————————————————————

"SHE," says she, entreated again by the wet snout.
Or, suddenly: "THAT."
Less than words
    emitted quivering in the ever-colder air
        where motes of dust float, or flecks of ash
            (sun very low, fire, shadows closing in)

———————————————————————

"She"…
Did I suggest: "the dog?"

..."She," she repeats, annoyed, "that."
She heard the word that I said, but ignores me.

Gathered up in this void,
she must, from minute to minute,
worry about this small... what?... presence? sustain it...
where?
"Her" focus more than dog-flesh pulsating halo
she tends to it with half-words that she chews (verbal scraps and sensations)
into a saliva paste

under her weak but obstinate gums
doubts and certainties become equal in a vital, milky continuity
for "her" for
"that."

She whispers: "her," "that," HER HER MMM
        she feeds it with the continuity of her throat and saliva sap

    THE SMALL PRESENCE that yes her IN OUT

... do I then feel poles of
identities gravitate materialize lunar blues
        in the early March evening

do her breaths (chch, mm) suspend positions and relations

depending on her — "her"
FOR THE LINK TO THAT...?

Pale, the night, through the small window-pane above us.
She murmurs, she hums.

———————————————————————

Is she making me (without meaning to, of course) enter for a second into the as-if of stories

as when in the shabby second-floor apartment
      time was condensed by the war, the snow,

        and everything behind the plane-trees' foliage, between those walls, despite the anxiety, was a game?

———————————————————————

… metamorphosis beating …

even if she barely speaks anymore, and seems
      only able at this point
          to pant — isn't it
              rhythmically, with very brief effects?
… and could it be that through her murmurs the composure of everything … changes and that every gap fills itself up — with what silky substance, what mud made of realization-mutability?

———————————————————————

She dozes, lit up by the dwindling fire.
The dog has gone to sleep, curled up on her lap.
Has everything lightened?

_____
_____

_____
_____

Cries — of night birds. FEET on the roof suddenly dance.

She wakes up. She may have only slept a quarter of an hour.

How feverish her drooping face is
and bitter her mouth!
   The dog stretches.

Here is
  (this is what I wanted — thought I wanted? — to get to...)

what she
tells me
  (me?
  no: this was it then, once and for all,
  no more stories addressed to me or whomever)

passionately,
though with a barely audible voice

    to listen to her continuously
      (to her who speaks not to me but to the void),
    is it to feel erasable that I need?

    I set my eyes on (hanging loose from one of the plaster walls) a
      light-bulb, its cold gleam (pressure...)

that she saw her, "HER," thus,
not leaping around anymore, but...

…how sad she was! she moans…

I saw her, says she
           (not to me: into the void)
lie down, yes,
no,
DROP DOWN on the threshold of the school.

———————————————————————

"She," lying down,
on the stone
body spread out — having suffered, "she," "that," brutally humiliated,
what refusal? rejection? —

*panting, in pain, wheezing
at the entrance of the courtyard
    thus, probably, on top of
        a rough piece of limestone
           (scrap of an orange-gray cliff) (mosses, grasses)…*

———————————————————————

*Yes yes
it's there*   she mutters
      (she hammers in a hushed voice, fingers bouncing
      opaque angry phrases off the dog)

it's from there
      (blazes on the brick chimney walls)
      now she's indignant in the darkness

*that "she"
was looking.*

Seated (old armchair), it's while looking at the fire
that she

       … sees? believes she sees?
feels and says *(the one thanks to the other)*,

that she forms in the void what "she"
      (at which point?)
saw
      from the threshold where she was lying, head on the stone,
      whimpering,
        at the back of the courtyard,

what for "her" (like long ago for her?) could,
over there, through the trees,

burn shine PROMISE…

―――――――――――――――

… *light of the sole classroom* —

I try to discern (understand-feel)
— as much as through her bits of sentences,
  by way of eclipses, breathings *(oh, ah, mmm)* (wonder, indignation, sadness) tossed off
into the darkness —

what it is *(now?)*, what it was *(long ago)* or could be

      FOR "HER"? HER?

to believe that she sees it...

concentrating under the linden trees,
infusing, so certain,
burning?

BUT WHAT WAS THERE ALSO, in that light,
that was false,
that was necessarily mean?

> *Glowing ambiguously,*
> *it, the light, waited, it had to wait*
> *(limpid yellow brew of insect wings, of*
> *black grains)*
> *full of former sensations*
> *to get back to*
>
> *dryness of the page under the side of the hand*
> *or, crashing against the painted wood or the pane's glass,*
> *the fragrant, dazzling, crystalline*
> *colored chalks*
>
> *(or even — on an earth-colored*
> *wool skirt — motionless,*
> *dry leaf, gaze, a praying*
> *mantis)*

that she offered — or
refused.

To this promise shining there, received from where, having subsisted where, other, (too strong?)
(promise... you know...: "Jude!")

it is now finally,
in the barn's night

that she — so weak, lost, incapable of raising herself up from the armchair —
objects-produces
this mixed body beyond names,
"her,"
this real-unreal crucial flesh.

SHE WAS PUSHED AWAY,
      she cries with a low voice, straightening herself up a bit, with difficulty,
      mouth trembling, cheeks inflamed,
yes, they shut the door on her, which the children had just gone through
        excited (that she did not say),
        after having tumbled down the plateau's nearby paths,
        laughing, jostling,

How she had run, though!
      she cries out again (softly).

And now she was sitting there. The only one to sit there.

She, that, the dog? her, her. Yes, of course: that.

She weeps, wrinkled face lit up by the fire.

Her hands rise above the sleeping dog,

  move forward into the void,
  bony (hematomas)

  trembling, vehement,
  accusatory.

What is she searching for this time?

She whirs with this refusal that she says she had witnessed,
      that she sees, there…

And, lifting herself up a bit, as in a wave of protest, of worry…, of spite,

"they should…," she pants.

———————————————————————
———————————————————————

NOW she must gather HER ANGER
— for the last time —

abstract,
gray gasping in the air
against what?

She would need to amass the objects of her anger

    a thousand objects against which I know she raged
    but —
     enormous ('14, '39, skies aflame, exodus,
      Indochina, Algeria)
     or apparently ludicrous things
    (in the country, in the city or suburbs, on the
      roads) —
     of which she wanted to know nothing but her rage,

*which she'll have always thought it necessary
not to begin to understand
(so as not to take the least part in it)...*

in order to feel one last time, in a single blow, radiating
from them, piled up through them

toward her, against "her"

*that which
always seemed to her
to be discarding, striking down,
    sacrificing... stupidly? ignominiously?*

    *— more or less sovereign decisions
    (to die for or to live only according to)*

      *yet become (for her? for so many!)
grotesque, naked, bloody*

---

    *... I doubt in the darkness, in my own way, I resist...
embers, cold...*

---

    *for "her," for "that,"
    (springing forth, with the children,
      scents of grass, rustling of
        leaves)*

    *it is promise itself — light, over there,
      between the black branches, in the back
    of the courtyard —*

that suddenly disfigured itself
darting out refusal

or that, with "her," she found to be
    related
to everything she had always hated

or rather: she had just forced it, this
light, this promise, to appear
arbitrary

today ... there ...
for "her," for "that,"
for what she was giving form to
on the spot,
— mixed, human-animal,
grotesque ... —
to this end that whatever was coming in
this light-promise
    might manifest itself
with no further justification
in a pure wavering
(which she expressed by way of the briefest anger
and this very mixture,
re-chewing, brooding over the distinctions and positions,
the names, the nouns ...
defeated half-words, frothing therefore, foam
    — rage and doubt —
quasi visible in the sparkling
bloody night)

CLAUDE MOUCHARD

THEY NEVER TEACH THEM ANYTHING,
   she suddenly pronounces in a stunningly clear voice, THESE —

she tenses up as if under a blow,
she's bumped into differentiation again,

these...

they... (*she's begun to cry again, faintly,*
   fresh old tears playing at slipping,
     at shining with the fire)

   (*she re-mumbles for an instant*)

nobody wants (*she begins again firmly*)

she has to (*here exactly is what she said*)..., everybody wants her to always stay
AS SHE IS.
And yet
   she began again, quickly
     (*before anyone could hear her? no,*
     before — had it still been possible —
     hearing herself)

I am sure she could...
THAT — yes —
  those, yes, were her words
WOULD LEARN

THAT WOULD KNOW...

  And then interrupted breath, coughs and crumplings:

    stubble or feathers are growing in the throat,
    where her voice loses itself.

ENTANGLED

―――――――――――――――――――――――――――
―――――――――――――――――――――――――――

That was it —
she had groped more than enough…

YOU…, *she repeated — to the void.*

She went quiet (saying nothing almost)
        for months, for a few years, forever.

―――――――――――――――――――――――――――

SILENCE.
    She fell deeply asleep at last — mouth agape

The night.
But exposed to that blaze
       — for one or two hours —
I still was,
       undecided, losing edges,
the possibility, the substance
of other points of confusion
       in the air of the barn,
spots or zones of indistinction (minimal, muddy) returned from far away, or born there — blending
the human, the animal, or generations, or things, leaves, grasses

whatever…

―――――――――――――――――――――――――――

She hardly spoke again, ever.

Did her power or desire to speak have to be nearly erased

for this zone of intermixture to become once more
    — for her and (to a certain extent) beyond her, or beside her, bit by bit —

more real than anything?

———————————————————

…and smoke… and gray veils stirring…

———————————————————
———————————————————

WAS SHE SOMEBODY FROM THAT POINT ON? How?

The accent lingered

resisting the quasi-loss of speech it passed into the chant which little by little
she merely whispered

it did not cease to be that old small difference
capable of diluting itself
without disappearing
orange or nut-brown cloud flowers
lal lalie
losing itself in the flowing water of sounds

(WAS SOMEBODY STILL THERE?)
(in the shell of the bones, under the ear, the temple)

— and like never before — finally —
light!

Papers!

For Jean, for Daniel

Canary Islands ... Boats emerge from the night amidst searchlights. Then, on a dock, bodies reel, held up by men in plastic white gloves. Are there any dead left in the boats? (Corpses will probably be washed ashore. We'll see pictures of them.)
It was on *France 2*, Monday **September 2, 2006**. At a late hour, it's true. But who has not seen things like that? Photos, in *Le Monde*, in *Libération*, etc. And on the internet.

> *Everyone has seen,* everybody knows, etc. **What is the use,** here, of churning out sentences?
> (Or of copying them?)

In broad daylight (a little later, in the same *France 2* report), two men, teenagers rather, are walking on the dock. They were unloaded there a few weeks before. They have been able (the voice-over tells us) to remain there, hired as interpreters. One of them says: "had I known, I would have stayed in my Africa, over there, there was always someone..."

October 4, 2006: seen by happenstance on LCI,[1] a Canary Islands resident (who, the voice-over tells us, takes care of illegals — as a psychologist? *I only caught this in passing, I've forgotten, already*) suggests (*but should his very suspicion be suspected?*) that the country's authorities count on this flow of illegals to earn European aid. He also implies that those undocumented people will be exploited by construction companies — in the heart of the Canaries' tourism boom (along those beaches where — as other images show — bathers sometimes discover bodies cast off by the sea).

Ladders made of scraps of wood... of anything, absurd grapples, against, atop, barbed wire...
Late September 2005, or early October, there had been (so they said) the "assault" (what a word!) on the borders of **Ceuta et Melilla**, Spanish enclaves on African land.

Libération, March 27, 2006:
"The wire fences of Ceuta or the electronic barriers of the Canaries or elsewhere will not discourage all those for whom an illegal's misery in Europe beats rotting in a village without hope in Sahel or in the forgotten outskirts of some African megalopolis."

*What can
these bits (news, memories of news) gathered here
(and immediately detached from present times…: in a void)
trigger beyond our usual sighs (while turning off the TV):
"this should not" be happening…, this "shouldn't have…"?*

*The illegals, if they are nothing but the debris, in "our" present,
of a future where everything would be accounted for and everyone settled,
how **could "we" really
think about them?***

*Might the question of illegals be outdated
from the start?*

And again, and indefinitely:

"First are the eyes, crazed, frightened, wandering without finding what to latch on to in the whirlwind of new images. The arms, outstretched to get something to drink, again and again, and quench the bottomless thirst…"
Benoît Hopquin, Los Christianos, *Le Monde*, October 14, 2006

*These quotations, or others (how many others could there be!),
to transport them here, to have them received (by way of these rough sentences),
is that to feel-test **the attention** that they
will have supposed or attempted — **in what "us"** — to arouse*

*(following, of course, that which could only be counted on
by the "eyes," the "arms, outstretched")…?*

"Our" shores, "our" borders...

And further, elsewhere — where the treatment of illegal migrants is being "externalized"?

"The so-called asylum externalization projects began appearing in European debates at the end of 2002, referring to policies meant to delocalize, to camps placed outside the European Union, the processing of asylum requests as well as the reception of asylum seekers and refugees. Developed by European governments in collaboration with the Office of the UN High Commissioner for Refugees (HCR) and the European Commission, these projects aim to create 'special safety zones' in certain regions of the world (central Africa, the Middle East...) in order to keep the refugees concentrated there and avoid in this way their migration toward European countries."[2]

Resolve the problem of migrants where that of human rights will not be raised...?

"When the neighboring States, and then, more broadly, the 'partner' States (notably within cooperation, development aid and humanitarian assistance programs) are led to do the work of retaining, locking up and deporting migrants in transit, it is no longer asylum that is being externalized, but the repression and detention of migrants."

From Cairo — December 30, 2005 (special correspondent from *Le Monde*):
"It's as though a hurricane had struck Moustafa-Mahmoud Square, just a few yards from downtown Cairo, in the upscale, peaceful neighborhood of Mohandessin. The forced evacuation of 1,500 Sudanese refugees by Egyptian police, on the night of December 30th, has left at least 23 dead [10 children, 7 women and 6 men, it is specified later on — with '*all anonymous*' added] as well as an unknown number of wounded among the refugees, and transformed the square into a ravaged field."

In Cairo — where do they hide, the "lost boys of Africa?"
"Though the phrase has come to be used specifically for the young Sudanese separated from their family when fleeing the civil war in the 1990s (Caroline Moorehead, *Human Cargo*),[3] [...] Cairo is full of lost boys, though most are no longer boys now, but young men from Sierra Leone and Liberia, Ethiopia and Eritrea, Sudan, Guinea, the Ivory Coast, Rwanda and Burundi. Over the last ten years, they have come to Cairo by a hundred different paths, on foot, by ferry, in airplanes, by trucks and trains, by camel or horseback, believing that, for all its horror, life was still worth living, that Egypt would be the gateway to a future, and that their past as victims of the savagery of civil war and modern conflict was somehow their passport to that future."

PAPERS!

"OUR" SHORE, what is it becoming, and what is happening to
OUR "WITHIN," OUR "AMONG OURSELVES"
today

> ... *wholly different from a few years or decades ago?*
>
> ***Boats gliding out of the night*** *among search lights ... Then used*
> *by Vietnamese or Cambodians ...*
> *Those, some (= "we"?) would look for,*
> *extending a hand to them ...*
>
> *January 3, 1980: it's the date in the "diary of a Christian survivor" that "Kim"*
> *(who, just before the invasion of Phnom Penh by the Khmer Rouge,*
> *had finished his "dentistry studies"),*
> *having fled Cambodia, and finally found refuge in the Chanthabury camp (Thailand)*
> *wrote by hand, in French and in English*
> *in order to try to be admitted by the United States or France*
> *(journal that he ultimately left here, "at home" — where (in October 2006)*
> *I am copying, just as they are, two or three fragments):*
>
> *"[...] Despite fever, hunger and exhaustion,*
> *I was able to set out alone for two nights and 3 days*
> *across the flooded plain of November and forests*
> *in the strictly controlled border zones of Battambang province."*
> [But hunger, he explains, forces him to approach a village, where he is immediately arrested...]
> *"I know that a horrible, cruel death will await me very soon."*
> *"[...] I am being closely watched and followed, in an abandoned pagoda,*
> *with my section of little guerillas dressed in black.*
> *Around the country, this particular chief is known for his genocidal acts.*
> *Anyone crossing his path, dares not look at his face,*
> *bows low and yields the way with respect.*
> *Except for me, no prisoner handed over to him escapes death.*
> *Within the pagoda precinct I saw ditches,*
> *freshly filled with dirt stained with human blood [...]"*
>
> *... **Kim,** who came from a camp in Thailand, had been sheltered for a few days*
> *in a reception center in the southwest of France*

before being taken to Orléans,
here *(we had given our address in response to a call published by Libération),*
where he arrived, *limping heavily,*
skin and bones (with the neck of a baby bird smashed naked on a sidewalk),
and got *... at last*
to eat
(mixing in a frying pan on the range, in a bath of sizzling oil,
eggs, sardines, butter),
and so — thanks to those few months, here, with us —
to become (not without bitterness, not without moments overwhelmed by powerlessness)
a caretaker for the elderly ... for
pallid bluish crumpled bodies.

... we

I tell myself — where? at home? in which places in the city? at which moments of our lives?

what are "we" becoming —, month after month, under the impact of what is thrown at us by newspapers or television, or by the (massive furtive) presence of those who (across deserts, seas and mountains, barbed wire, threats and checks)
get here — get to "us"?

What do we metamorphose into in each of those cases where we claim that "we"
(our "among ourselves" — whose obviousness is obviously only an image at once peeled off,
flaking —,
our supposed "lifestyle,"
our rights — reserved for us? marks of what election?

are safe from the irruption
(or if we attempt to ignore it still)?

As with the pressing of an overly cool palm *(opaque-dazzling) on one's eyes,*
when does the "we," *in the streets, in the city's differentiated places*
(or in the whirling "between" gnawed again in the air),

slam down on my attention
— that of one who, non-migrant,
sedentary
will have for a whole lifetime stomped around these same places —

> *so as to open me wide, smash me again*
> **well short of** *myself*
> *— of that being-oneself with which, like anyone, I will have been burdened —*
> *and take me apart in the air in fickle spots of free receptivity*
> *that don't look back at themselves…?*

The "**WITHIN**," the "**WE**": to crudely **taste,** in the odor of the streets, on the bridge, at home (in the entrance, the hallway, the air that changes from one room to the next) **its ferrous flavor, its rippings, its violence?**

The warm reddish "**AMONG**," *re-exhaled everywhere from moving bodies, from faces as they project themselves on it,*
how to realize it as it reveals itself (yet fades again at once, formidable) **in the moments when** the effects of **its outer limit** (of its determination — or that of arranged access paths — by power) make themselves felt
or in the moments-places
where this very limit **passes through the middle**
that is to say
    always, presumably, by plugging itself, black fluid, into the "within's" inner divisions,
    its equivocations and reversals,
    but especially, violently, insolubly, today, **through the "illegals."**

In an "**ALL-SECURITY CITY**" like Orléans

> *where I try*
> *(at my home, yes, protected, certainly: ancient family core … doors, windows, walls (which have always, in truth [since the (world) war], seemed steeped in night) —*
> **to set these sentences**
> **without,** *perhaps,* **stopping**

CLAUDE MOUCHARD

their rehashing in the heart of the "within's"
own element

— a testing ground of sarkozysm, for many years now —

for example in the streets leading down to the Loire, which, ancient, narrow,
have been repaved whitened:
the making of a ferocious sheep's "we"
for which it was necessary to wash, off the walls, the life of time
(erasing the precious, decipherable — Balzacian — black-rusty layers)
and realize, irreversibly, the idiotic ideal whereby
every stone is disguised (as Deguy would more or less put it) as itself

how, in the very places where gazes are directed, could one not sense that one's own sensations are being followed by wakes
the furtive arrivals of those whom smugglers will have dropped here (rather than in Paris?), in the streets, in the middle of the night…

Chechens, two or three years ago, noticed
by members of one of those associations
which alone try to keep watch
(a resource that Sarkozy has undertaken to destroy)
as they were wandering in the darkness under the November rain…
H. goes…:
discussion on the spot — then, in the days and months to follow:
mediations, oppositions, compromises with institutions, etc.

*And **who were they, those glimpsed***
(by H. and me, while driving, by chance)
*one freezing night, **in the center of the city,***
between the museum and the cathedral,
and to whom (from a small truck) the Red Cross
itself embroiled (instrumentalized?) in what negotiations
with the "authorities" (the prefecture, whitish mass nearby?) —
was giving out soup…?

"They have to suffer," a secretary from the prefecture supposedly said, two or three years ago,
"So they won't get used to it." "So they won't attract others…"

ON THE EDGE OF THE LOIRE (south bank, maybe one or two kilometers east of the city), off the road,

in one of those muddled zones where an absence of checking seems to prevail (yet too far, this particular spot, from the city for there to be, as in other places of this kind, trafficking, deals, sexual among others)

willows, osiers, masses turning over in the wind, the current,
suddenly,
so bright (merging then with the sky),
high thickets,
strips of shifting sand,
fragrant Loire mud subtly colored and marvelously fine
(like that drawn from inside a clog
in which Andersen tale?)
and birds, rodents of all sizes

banks that one could see, at the end of the **forties**
(broken, collapsed bridge: slanted blocks, metal stems)
from long black boats

or, on a bicycle, some years later,
in the semi-darkness where the paths vanished,
to feel (the ground rolling out in the halo of headlights) the real
crackling with maybes
or (grainy ocher power of the continuous)
emerge from itself in amazing myriads of intermediaries

— where we (H. and I) had been summoned one Sunday morning (in which cold early Spring ?), by G., the correspondent from *Le Monde* in Orléans, not far from a facility where elderly North Africans without family
live in retirement —

how many are there, who have sought refuge — illegals —
and crammed themselves, at night, in narrow concrete shacks (probably abandoned working-class garden sheds)?
Most are **looking at us,** standing, **silently** …

Living there — we learn this without having asked for identities or origins — are a few Algerians, one Egyptian, Africans (there is only one woman, staying — they open one of the sheds to show us … mattresses and blankets in a heap … — with one of the men).
And (through the Egyptian) a few young men from Darfur make themselves known.

We wander around a little (plastic bags and bottles strewn in the brush, inevitably, papers, rotten mattresses) … admittedly without demanding to see everything.

No faucet, we notice.
The one which could have been used, by the road, a few hundred meters from there, has been shut off it seems — on which authority's request? by what decision to dissuade them from staying?
What do they drink? What they receive, along with food, from association activists.

> In Nanterre's gigantic slum, back in the years '60–'61,
> on the side of a "national" highway (Sunday evening cars),
> (fields of mud without any equipment, shacks made of debris, bits of planks, cardboard, sheet metal and fabric)
> (and also: [contradictory] threats, inspections … curfew, gun shots, in the night, with "real bullets")
>
> it was, for the children
> a long trek
> to the sole accessible water source
> — just beyond "their" space, beyond that "among," despite everything, crudely,
> constituted there —

small carts
with big wheels dragged and pushed through the reeking ruts
and heavy aluminum containers
(salvaged from antiquated "Arab" grocery stores)

To wash themselves (and their clothes), they have the water of the Loire:
"we…" (an Algerian man is translating for us — though he admits having trouble understanding the Arabic of people from Darfur), "we smell bad"…
and they have us, indeed, smell, not without expressing, with gestures, their humiliation, the sourness exhaling from the folds of their clothes steeped in particles of mud
(that mud which — on the water's gliding, gyrating surfaces or in the whirlpools and despite suddenly white wrenchings — is turning the river brown.)

As we get back in the car, two of the youngest, sitting on a kilometer marker by the highway, expressively follow us with their eyes.
Since they seem to have been waiting for us there, we walk toward them (and others then also come closer, chime in, translate a little more, awkwardly).
One of the two complains of fever, of head pains. The other rolls up a sleeve, shows his forearm: little bumps everywhere, I feel them with my fingertip. Scabies?

"A resurgence of diseases!"
"tuberculosis, scabies"
(Words from the Orléans deputy mayor in charge of public safety)

It's a Sunday afternoon, and the hospital, where we take them, refuses — politely — to examine them.

At the office of a doctor on call (in a suburb), the waiting room is full: women with little children (ear infections).

We wait.
With one of the two,
who speaks a little English (learned, he says, by listening to the radio),
I go back to the hallway:

his father, a livestock farmer, was (he explains, groping for words) killed
and his mother (after militias had ordered him to join them
or be shot)
urged him to flee
(leaving her alone with his sisters).

And then… the five of us (the two of them, G., H., and I) enter the examination room.
The doctor, young, visibly exhausted (kids shouting), protests ("this isn't a lounge"),
expresses (as soon as he understands that the two fall under the CMU) his
bad mood (without going so far, like
others, as to refuse to examine them) and after a few sentences
that will have been enough to soften him, he auscultates, palpates, writes out prescriptions.

And, of course, there will follow (days, weeks, months even)
many more episodes, pharmacy, laundry, money, etc.
then … other interventions,
including, finally, one — worrisome —
from the administration …

*("**There are some!**"*
It's a nurse shouting — in the world of the Kolyma, where Shalamov
survives among hundreds of thousands of zeks.
"'There are some, Lidia Ivanovna!' he said
and screamed at Andreev: 'Why are you covered with lice, huh?'
But the doctor did not let him go on.
'Is it their fault?' she said quietly and in a tone full of reproach,
stressing the word 'their,' and she took her stethoscope from the table.") [4]

A few weeks later, we will learn
that two of these men (from Darfur), returning from the city toward "their"
bank of the Loire, and crossing the tracks of the railroad bridge in the dark,
were run over.

PAPERS!

> (The short item in the local newspaper mentioned that the "papers" of one of them had been recovered..., and that his family had supposedly been told [?])

Le Monde, October 11, 2006 (from the Nairobi correspondent):
"In Darfur, the Ramadan truce is over. While the Sudanese government, for the last three months, has amassed troops in this region, as vast as France, of the country's Western part and recruited new militias, a major offensive against the rebels and the population of Darfur seems imminent.
[...]
An account of the extreme violence routine in Darfur was published Monday by the office of the United Nations High Commissioner for Human Rights, describing a series of attacks against the village of Buram, in Southern Darfur, between August 28 and September 1. The attack, led by militias recruited within the 'Arab' tribes by the Sudanese security forces, is said to have left hundreds of civilians dead. No rebel, it seems, was present in Buram. The United Nations are underscoring the responsibility of the Sudanese government for this massacre, even as it requests that an investigation be carried out to identify the perpetrators."

TO LET ONESELF BE STOPPED or rather
TO BE ("us") INTERRUPTED — by what comes from the edge, or from beyond the edge..., by what happens to suddenly pass through the middle of the "within"?
To be able to be interrupted: generosity, liberty...?

Still, **in order to live with irruptions**

from phone calls at any hour, email alerts...
or simply: **by accepting,** *in the street, on TV,* **to see**
what one did not plan to see,
— and in such a way, if possible, **as to**
draw consequences...

mustn't one **be continuous enough,**
sufficiently equipped with strength
not to fear to be exposed to them?

For interruptions from poverty are entirely sterile: nothing
but entanglements of lives muddled from then on
(shouts, passages hurtling through, musics cutting each other off, defiant signals, ads,
endless claims, insults)

nothing but (unstable, nervous) impossibility to form lasting aims
... nothing except powerlessness
(or even, soon — multiplying hatreds...)

Is it only for those who are **here by right**
in the element (however equivocal) of the "within,"
that it is permitted
(right? happiness? anxiety?)
to be interrupted by that which
(those who)
will find itself *(themselves)*
bursting in,
smashing (for one infra-second) any aim...
like, through foliage,
sprays, splashes...
psychic blood

BLUE simply, ashy, apparently calm, around 6 pm (November ?)
The Post Office **SQUARE**

(an almost central place, but a little removed within the city)
(a street starts from there where Blacks, Turks, gather more and more) (the municipality seems to be plotting to push them further away...)

renovated maybe thirty years ago, a large drab building

as though transparent
for someone born like me during the war:
the memory still throbs of a color, happy-acid one, that of the massive brick cube
that the Post Office still was after the war, having survived the bombings of '44
— not far from heaps of white ruins, guttings of the city down to its cellars
(green pools of water, in the rubble under the open sky, for years)

In the middle, a stretch of ugly lawn, synthetic slabs, a tramway line, a few benches. Sweetness — with what metallic taste?

> *On the other side of the square, Social Security, a few benches, elderly North African men (at certain times)…*

The Post Office (court of wet shiny gray vaguely orangy synthetic slabs) is not yet closed (light through glass doors)
Blacks, Africans — probably — (quite a few women, children chasing pigeons) are assembled there, in small groups, in the autumn cold…

I'm coming out of a warm, small travel agency where I got a ticket for the United States.

Papers, mine (passport, this time, with a work visa, letter on onion skin paper, et cetera: "documents" — objects of slightly feverish care — mixing, in my pockets, their odor with that of clothes, of sweat).
Papers, theirs. "Theirs"? I have no reason to assume, in fact, that they are all in equivalent situations. Be this as it may, the post office (the counter) is for everyone the place for savings, for money orders; it's the link that connects them with over there…

> ***On one edge** of the square, **a tramway** has stopped in the slowly gathered darkness, it **takes off again** (to dive into several kilometers of suburbs) lit from within, bodies crammed in, elbow to elbow, face to face — making sure to ignore one another. If **some quasi-attention** runs through nonetheless (which each face, as though lapped by a flame's reflection, may fleetingly receive) it's not for one another but **for what**, among them all, cannot be fully contained and **burns**.*

"I SHOULD NOT BE HERE"
(here — outside of every "within"...?)

> It's mistakenly, of course
> (aggregating, by a very common, facilitating foolishness, too many "others" in clumps,
> where
> in fact distinctions are vital),
> that, day-dreaming (sheltered), **I will have**, for a moment,
> while reading a little later (thus at home) Judith Soussan[5]
> (her book discovered on the internet accompanies me, at least intermittently),
> **attributed that voice
> randomly to one** of those whom I tried to make myself picture again
> (though already too mixed up in my memory)
> as they were — **on the Post Office square.**

"I should not be here..." That remark was made by Désiré, a homeless African. It was therefore collected in *Les SDF africains en France*.

Judith Soussan listened, transcribed, and among her reflections, she welcomes, in her own way, such words from people who are "on the margins."
"Those 'margins,'" she calmly notes, "can enlighten us."

"**... Because it's open inside my head and I don't know what to take...**"
Those particular words, transcribed elsewhere in the book,[6] are spoken by another homeless African: Cyprien.

To take something — that which one can hold on to in spite of everything, an idea to orient one's life — from inside one's head?

If **"it's open,"** does Cyprien still have an **"inside"** in his head?
His head (so the reader of Cyprien's remarks will think), perhaps it is open because he has **nothing within which to be,** because **nothing envelops him.**

In order to be capable of seizing one's own thoughts — or perhaps even just one's sensations and emotions, one's desires, or a modicum of hope — is it necessary to be **within** something?

Is it thus necessary to belong, can one only relate to oneself by knowing that one is contained within?

A single "within"?
or several concentric "withins," reinforcing one another
(*orbs of heat reddening, for whose sixth sense, the streets' air?*)

or complex, intersected, proving incoherent?
*even incompatible, to the point of madness,
of vibrating, of mutual breaking
(like envelopes made of glass, in the void,
absurd, bloody edges)*

To be — to know — to identity oneself… as what? homeless? without papers?
Cyprien (heard by Judith Soussan): "I couldn't even feel myself in there."

Judith Soussan pays attention to what distinguishes itself, even opposes itself, within those margins hardly seen by most of "us."
Further, she gives access to what each speaker attempts to think about where they are…

Nuances in (sociological? administrative? judicial?) categorizations…
Or rather, between the homeless and the undocumented: difference between economic and political characterizations, respectively? or (equally) between that for which one could be held responsible and that for which one cannot possibly blame oneself?

Cyprien: "This didn't bother me at all, because it's what I didn't want, there was only one thing blocking me, that was papers, and for me it wasn't my fault."
And he insists: "There was no feeling of guilt… I didn't feel implicated."

> *(Why did he note, in passing: "Before the term 'undocumented,' it was*
> *'aliens without proper legal status'?")*

Cyprien: what is it to have one's head open and to feel its "content" losing itself in the void — in tiny dots, which, neither within nor without, sizzle, scatter?

Where, in which place (the street, a square perhaps *like that of the Post Office*, the bank of a river, a squat),
to be able only to feed, with all of one's strength,
a hemorrhage of blinding points:
nothing but micro-palpitations of the incomprehensible, while time vanishes?

Within what to think, in the evening, while going to sleep — **or in the morning**, while going where…?

But Cyprien or Désiré (fed, clothed, sheltered)…, at least "belong" to that minimal "within" which Emmaüs would like to constitute.

Press Release (Paris, March 22, 2006)
"[…] The Emmaüs France movement, which encompasses more than 250 structures for shelter and assistance to people in trouble, expresses its strong reservations regarding the draft legislation of February 9 modifying the CESEDA (Code of Asylum Rights and of Entry and Stay for Foreigners), as well as the February 21 memorandum entitled 'Conditions for the arrest of an alien without proper legal status, detention of aliens without proper legal status, penal responses,' distributed to prefects by the Ministry of the Interior.
The Emmaüs groups welcome an average 20% to 25% of foreigners in their midst. They consider the act of welcoming all people with the same rights and duties, and without any criteria for selection at entry, to be two fundamental requisites of their integration and of the development of their abilities."

The "Within" itself: meant to be sensed (savage taste) — where? when? by or for whom?

To sense it in the raw instants that reveal it as the torn,
threatening, condition
of feeling itself...

> *...with, always, the imminence*
> *of its possible destruction*
> *(like long ago, in wartime, houses with blue panes,*
> *vibrations under a sky invaded*
> *by monstrous objects)*

To feel oneself belonging, and as though infused by the "within"?

special sheen (for example in airports)
— suddenly dangerous? —
of those who, even when away from "home" (trade, tourism),
fall under a protective state,
who, without thinking about it,
sense this at every moment

Is it to comply with, believe in something politically decided — something circumscribing (containing) and excluding?

> Would a political society be something to experience
> as a "complete and closed social system"?
> "It is complete in that it is self-sufficient
> and has a place for all the main purposes of life.
> It is also closed [...] in that entry into it is only
> by birth and exit from it is only by death." (Rawls)[7]
>
> Yet Lefort:
> "... it would not be appropriate to locate man 'within' society ..."[8]

To im-migrate: to pass — feel oneself pass (presume to be seen passing) — within what?

Within what common visibility — here, in Orléans, for example — would one know one is known about? with hostility? or try to remain unknown?

Within what implicit and powerful element (the powdery availability of the "between") would one hope to be taken into account? Succeed, count, leave a mark — or, by moving forward, possibilize the air itself?

But, even while risking **here** (hoping, fearing) a new visibility (to administrators, or in people's gazes-ideas),
desperately, at great cost (to the point of exhaustion), strive to never stop counting — and be quasi-visible, imagined, hoped for —
in the eyes of those who stayed **over there** (and who wait, need, count on...)

To have (intrepid? overwhelmed?) to live (not, at times, without cockiness and pretense, or, alas, to the point of bitterness... years, fatigue, fall) within **two "withins"** (...linked by wire transfers, telephone calls)?

What do we know (feel-think), "we" (assured of our places inside one — several? — "withins"),
of "their" reasons to leave?

"The spiral of rejection [*who is speaking here? I lost... copied from the internet then lost... it comes from* Cultures et conflits][9] begins with a story: the asylum seeker tells what led him to leave his country and this written or oral account is difficult and, necessarily, long..."
"Even the explanation of a hurried departure must go over several years of life: either because the exile's situation has insidiously deteriorated down to a stage, subjectively felt, of crippling fear; or because the triggering factor however rapid doesn't spare the exile an ulterior need to go far back into time to explain to himself, first, and to others afterwards, this strange overturning in his life; or finally because the chaotic society that pushes one into exile conceals a complexity that is difficult to master [...]"

"… the asylum procedure forms leave no room for this kind of expansion […]. The rejections are massive, the procedure is expeditious and inquisitorial. The petitioner first exposes himself in writing and in a few pages. The narrative is brief, dry, improvised on a counter corner, under the pressure of the line behind, handicapped by its reliance on an intermediary […]."
"Then come the hearing stages," "the same observation of a collision between the time allotted for listening and the possibility for the exile to make himself understood."

Who, among us (and, supposedly, "for us"), listens to these words? Administrative oversight (hence papers, files, reports, surveillance, arrests, expulsions)

Who, among us (for us?) tries to perceive and analyze this
listening? "Scientifically"? Politically?
(hence articles, books, media programs, interventions — sometimes —)

Who is watching? Who is watching the watching?
Nearly identical individuals, whose trainings have to be closely related —
but between whom it happens that every "we" must be torn.

WHO, AMONG US, WHAT, WITHIN US, through ourselves or others,
WHAT WE-ATTENTION, WHAT GAZE-INSTANCE,

was presupposed, hoped for,
looked for

which "we"
standing for a powerful other
that would be wished for (demanded — to the point, sometimes, of hating it)
by hundreds of thousands of abandoned people?

by this TV report

> — which, at the same time it knows
> how to find what it shows us, digs for our sake (anticipating it)…
> at whose initiative (and with what prior information)
> was the project conceived, and with what means, granted by whom, was it created?

on child-slaves in Ghana, bought by fishermen, five or six years old, barely fed, in rags, beaten…?

One (having noticed that others were bought back by an association and that he could not be) is seen crying,
from the side, his face against the lake,

seen more than alone, and yet, there, this one time, for sure, **aware that he is being seen, having, therefore, felt himself,** but for how many minutes, **known about**

then — what?

> And for those "bought back," what do we glimpse of their parents
> — by whom they (less abandoned little tom thumbs than
> negotiable bodies)
> will very likely be resold?
> *(A false — premature — old man, toothless, laughing,*
> *in the middle of what doesn't manage to be a village,*
> *boasts*
> *of having fathered twenty children and sold five.)*

> And, of those who buy them,
> what do we see?

PAPERS!

A long thin woman's arm sticks out from behind a canvas
(at a market),
grabs a child, pulls him away from "our" gazes:
"this child is mine!,"
"she's lying," the guide-interpreter whispers (a local man,
vaguely sneering),
"it's a child-slave."

From where, and when, for "us" (in the distance or in the city already), **will it again burst forth,** unexpected, obsessive,
the question

that **of the edge**
irrupting, thunderbolt tasting of ink,
in the middle …
dismantling every realization of **our supposed "within,"**

finding it suddenly where, burning, it
can no longer be contained within itself …,

from which angle will it shoot out again,
from which corners or folds
of the outside-within,

from what knots of problems and solutions in need of maintenance
(such as where, right at noon,
on Martroi Square, among banks, the chamber of commerce, cafés,
in a demonstration for the
undocumented where members — nearly a hundred —

were gathered from various associations, PTA, etc.,
H., going from one to the next,
secured a hiring promise for M. O., a Congolese man seeking papers
or rekindled from
what nasty bucklings of intervisibility
(those places or minutes where certain people, in broad daylight,
are imperceptible or, on the contrary,
cruelly fail to not be seen:
that man, for instance, delivered — in a lit tramway station (10 pm) we
pass by — into the hands of the police (who handcuff him)
by an agent who noticed that he was lacking not only a
"ticket" but papers…
…a woman (fifty years old?) drunk or crazy, or simply at the end of her rope…,
kicked off the tramway and punished with a fine,
shouts from the edge of the sidewalk, begs that they let the man go (she does not know him),
hooting sobs and curses…
And us (H. and I)? We become concerned, we insert ourselves, inquire, pester…:
"if you want to know what's going on," says one of the cops, "join the police…"

TO SAY-ACTUALIZE FOR AN INSTANT — the "we," the "within" itself: only sentences could do that whose necessity (shaping impulse) **would always be reborn through an eruption from inside or outside, from what furrows this "within" with darkness,** criss-crosses it with a fluidity, a freshness altogether too raw,

sentences unwinding black-porous soaking up all attention,

self-devouring formulations imposed by the instants-places where, right in the heart of "within," something

non-envelopable is being recreated, because of the perennially recreated divisions, those of the too far-too near, those of inner linings inflamed with incompatibility, or of something **non-appropriable,** necessarily disputed among many, in a game that proves too serious, rippings that soon turn bloody,

but also, inextricably, something **disputed between self and self,** some time-substance-self unfolding through changes of states (from the "ordinary" to what excitements, rages, sexual faintings, feral places-moments of bodies), or made rugged by absorptions (passions, absolute dependencies), by highs and lows (incontrollable jolts of feeling, mismatches and blackish collapses of thoughts)

and further, surreptitious, continuous, radiant, vitally scented and dripping with sap: contacts, **flesh-thing alloys,** alliances or supports (humans, plants, animals, etc. — all this always on the verge of crushing itself, catastrophic…)

LIVING (visible? invisible?) IN THE EDGE, in the very thickness of the edge
LAURA (about thirty, two children)?

>   (**Why did she flee Angola?** She thought she explained that to
>   various bodies…
>   In one case, the last almost, H. was present; the members of that appeal board seemed
>   shaken…, moved!
>   H., returning, had said she was nearly certain of a positive decision at last…
>   And then — rejection. So as to stick to the quotas set by the ministry?)

Laura, then,
several months ago, separated for a while from her children
(for caution's sake),
had been sheltered ("protected") here, "at home"

>   (until, defended, claimed as it were, against the prefecture, by a UDF[10] mayor
>   from the suburbs, she was housed in a building of the psychiatric hospital on the edge of
>   the forest and finally received papers — temporary ones, to be sure)

and I tried, talking, to make her forget her anguish

>   (hands writhing, whitened lips:
>   for fear of the "DDASS"[11] which, she cried,
>   was going to "take" her six-year-old boy and her four-year-old girl)

thus she told me how she had at times
(because she had to leave in the morning the emergency shelter where she had found refuge)
spent, with her daughter (while the boy was at school),
hours, in winter, **in the well-lit warmth surrounding a** huge **"megastore"**

>   (the only one that has been allowed — through what "influences"? — to set itself up
>   in the center of Orléans),

>   without, then, entering the store itself (how to pay for anything at all?),
>   but restricting herself to the proximity of the cash registers (where, highly visible, in white
>   shirts, security guards stand around — mostly black…)
>   wearing down the hours, with her little girl,
>   sheltered, both of them, though on the very edge, by that metallic whale's carcass…

        and she was not the only one, she explained to me…
   others were wandering there, silent (except when there was trouble)

     she, like all those marginalized, being **visible**, of course, but **without being**
          (out of tolerance? counting for nothing in the cameras' eyes?) **seen,**
                        right **on the edge**
              of this very poor **palace of visibility**
                (the one that products compete for:
    wrappings — cardboard boxes, plastic, cellophane — calculated colors, contacts,
   smells of "clean," sickly sweet, or acid, or oil as though pleated into the ridges of bottles
              products sparkling with emulation to appear exactly "made for"
      ("for," one minute, whatever gang of young girls, supple gleaming giggling avid, as much as for
                    things, for their own intervisibility in the cash register lines),
           and become ever more completely what would forever be expected
                   like sugar dissolving, perfect, without residue,
                             in the night of taste

And him again, IN HIS HEAD,
what could he possibly have,
        what in the world could he "tell himself,"

this guy, rue de la République?

                                        but me, just as well,
          at that moment (half-running) was I formulating sentences **in my head?**

                          …half-words, maybe, yes, a froth
          of enthusiasm under the spell of the horizontal sun on the Loire
                slate-grey heron hunched in the cold,
           egret — dazzling-dazzled in the light? —
      emerging with wary but suddenly quickening steps,
          out of yellowed tufts trapped in ice…
                  ("for" no one,
            those lives excitedly caught
          like a sexual secret of "nature"?)

He was there, this November morning (right on my way to the station), black man (of unclear age),
standing in the middle of the street

> (the one with the most shops, the only one downtown haunted by kids from the outskirts)

frozen man

come out of where in the near dawn?

> *oddly,*
> *he had not (not yet? it was barely daybreak)*
> *been prohibited from being there*
> *— despite all the decrees passed in Orléans*
> *so that no one encounter anything but*
> *the expected*

so where did he fall from, and how?
it was shortly after the riots, the stone-throwings:
canceled trams and night buses, chaos, perhaps intended, of communications with the suburbs

The previous summer,
I had spotted him several times, in this same street, wandering in the crowd, stopping at length, or seated, sometimes, on a tram-stop bench, carrying ragged packages, poorly tied, downy-excoriated,
in the sun, among a bunch of teens (nonchalant, or shot through with waves of excitement)

once he had seemed to me (not far from FNAC,[12] in front of a clothing store) to have struck up, confusedly, a conversation with some of them)
Blacks? Beurs?[13] also some of those translucid blonds from the north (descending from Polish immigrants?),

> most dressed in a coded manner, of course, but one not unable to surprise, jump out…
> they weren't jeering — not really…
> incredulous rather, interrupted in their hunger to see, to be seen,
> they seemed stupefied instead, or worried
> — on this edge of visibility

less than thirty, probably — long woolly brownish black locks (self-braided for lack of care, or the remains of an elaborate hairdo…)

> ***describe*** him?
> *give him, here, the attention he was destroying?*

now standing in the barely risen day, in the freezing wind of a crossroad,

motionless stiff (no longer capable of sitting) in the middle of scurrying people (each one running within his own anticipated visibility, that of a day to live through)

blunt stern planted in the middle of the flux

his packages (the same ones from the summer?) piled up near him
> (under the feet, almost,
> of those who suddenly discovered them on the gray stone pavement)

a soaking wet loaf of bread, tied to the side of one of the bundles, and sticking out in the way

and **he pyramid-like**
as though made of the folds of torn transparent plastic in which he had tried to wrap himself, or of the overflowing layers-crusts of his random, superimposed clothes
some magnificent glimpsed vestiges, bits of what cast-offs…
leather, dazzling swatches of fabric, pieces gathered from where? for
theatrical brocades, for the hallucinatory display of a rotting self

so many humid **heaps** against the cold, or against… what?
apotropaic like shouts? like wringings of hands? in the void

and beneath, what hard-to-imagine body? in what state?
and **in**
his head? what?
what words waiting? or ... half-words

> was he ... making himself, still, promises to "pull myself through," could he
> still tell himself that he was *not*
> what he was
> there ...

> *(and what if one morning it had been one of my children, discovered there, and such, at*
> *the end of such a night — that ...)*

he didn't extend his hand
hadn't next to him, like others (that beggar woman — Asian, exceptionally — always on the same threshold,
a bit further on, but at other hours), **a plastic cup** where he might have put a few coins to prime the giving

and ... at the moment when I

> **tell that story?**
> to have believed I could, childishly, bring that home ...

bump into his packages, he coughs, a face from which water wrings, spits out

did I get splashed — and ... worried ... — about being soiled? contaminated?

no sooner have I passed him than I can't — *hooked by what, and harshly brought back?* —
but turn around and (looking for a coin in my pocket)
address him: "you ... you need ...?" "some ...?"

his lids semi-sealed stuck with secretions painfully part, exposing the white (beneath the
irises) of half-rolled-up globes

from his lips a faint wheeze — a laugh?

he drips he steams *condensing-decomposing the air between our faces*
he exhales the thawing of the fog that, all night long, had frozen on him

halo of ammonia
from the urine that broke through his wrappings,
drool on the fleecy beard

I touch his hand suddenly (without him saying a word) visible

what then (fear for a second)
*if **that hand then** grabbed me*
(in the moment when i'm going to catch "my train")
and if suddenly there
were to imperiously materialize the link
which we always knew could — should? — be created with the one to whom we gave,
a formidable (devouring?) dependency

but
now, here, well — I…
got a bit lost, I let go

I no longer know what, at this point, I should have articulated, which details…
nor why

this man — more than alone, "disaffiliated" —, was he necessarily **undocumented?**

homeless, yes, illegal, maybe not

distinctions between situations can be decisive
and above all (Judith Soussan) vital "inside" a "head,"
the head, there, of this frozen man,
during, especially, those hours where maybe he tried to… "speak to himself"
— in the middle of the street that morning —

absorbed in maintaining his continuity
— "within"? "without"?

> and so if..., in these sentences, I was tending toward
> a political argument, have I just lost it,
> and haven't I simply drowned it back in
> whatever reimposed itself, submerging, from the half-thought sensations
> of the street?

I saw him again once more in December in front of the Post Office
(at some distance from the groups of Africans)

> leaning back, one evening, on the wall, just one bundle, a whitish roll (to sleep on?),
> stuck behind him,
> he was playing a reed-pipe (found where?)
> tapping, on the flat stones of the square still lit by the lingering day,
> with one foot
> without seeming to see anyone
> gazeless
>
> holding a coin in my hand I gave him, from the top of my arm,
> a slight nudge
> from the side
> and again his hand, barely, came out
> and I brushed his fingers of
> chapped brown-orange leather

then never again

OR AGAIN, *but quickly, it's too late (time has run out)*

LIKE A KNOCK ON (or a **grip on**) **THE SHOULDER**,
forcing me to turn around toward what was happening, behind me, at Roissy, as I had just passed through — glass booths — document controls
in a hurry, like everyone else, to separate myself from the mass of passengers from the same plane,

what took hold of me?

This was (returning from Beijing, a few colleagues who had exited before me waving goodbye from afar already)
not exactly, for sure, **a matter of no papers,**
but rather one of insufficient papers … [?],

enough to block there
he who, during the flight, had been my companion

> for eleven hours
> I had been seated — among Chinese passengers exclusively,
> who seemed more or less organized in a group
> *(naive, perhaps, what was I not seeing?)* —
> next to him
>
> my neighbor to the left (window side)
> (stiff brown jacket, round hands, thick pock-marked face)
> *at meal time (on Air France),*
> *his bread, which he does not know how to put in his mouth,*
> *I show him how to break it, etc.*
> **(*fraternization!*)**

but I cannot now … express, release that grip (it will never cease to hold me)

simply, **it was then,**
— worried (my own body revolted) about him (stopped there as I was going through), imagining his forced return, the money (whose …? lost), the mess and (family, village) the humiliation —

it was …,
turning around toward the cop, against him,
almost taking "action" (pointless? or worse?)
crying out for real — and yet as in a dream (waking surrounded by all in the process of realizing one's nightmare)!

Will I "come back" to it? **Nothing,** here, obviously — not the piercing evidence, not the confusion, or blindness, **nor**
the question:
nothing has subsided, **nothing stops — there**

Notes

From Darfur to the Loire with Ousmane to begin

> Who asks your opinion of this stranger?
> And if you give it without having being asked,
> go then night after night
> with his sores on your feet, go on, and don't come back.
> Ingeborg Bachmann[14]

"come on": he makes a cutting gesture with his hand in the white air.
For months now, on a regular basis, we have been talking — in the kitchen usually. Have I made him believe that on top of the three or four years of deprivation he has recently gone through we would be able, as long as he is living with us and we take the time we need, to lay down words day after day, like the soothing fold of a blanket?

"Come on, get going." With his earthy-bitter voice, and his arm (dark silhouette against the light), he mimes those who free you or chase you away. In a street, back then, in Libya. Or, after an overnight police custody, in a street of Paris or Orléans. Or at the door of a detention center, by a road in the Orléans forest, miles away from anything ("What do I do?" he asked the policeman. "Not my problem… Come on, get going.")

"Come on, get…" He expels into the air sentences that, for months, have stayed implanted in him like stings.

But suddenly, it is he who, standing in front of the glowing glass door, facing me, addresses these words to himself: **"Come on, get going."**

"Get going…" He has nowhere to go, except to this family of "whites" (as he said to me), this house where he has been living for nearly a year now, this kitchen…
Have we given him false hopes? Papers, a job: his or our helplessness — administratively maintained — is too likely to become final.

"Here," he says, plunking himself down again in the chair, **"this is not a life"** — or (I'm transcribing) **"not-my-a-life."**

"**Claude,**" he says, looking at the gray tiles, "**I'm going to leave.**" Where for? To risk disappearing in a Khartoum prison? Or, if he gets out after several months, to try to find his vanished mother and sisters... or, perhaps, only the devastated site of his village, or the remnants of his house?

"**Here,**" he hammers — and I'll have nothing to answer —, "**this is not-my-a-life.**"

*

Words of Ousmane — or "O." — an exile from Darfur...
Why did I begin with those — among so many others, which I have been hearing from his mouth for almost a year now, and which I keep (as I'm completing these very lines) hearing still?

He had said them weeks ago... But until now they had remained suspended in the air — imminent. It's only very recently — **May 20, 2008** — that I decided to write them down — or, by my hands, to let them strike, pitch-black.

*

Jot down what O. says, for the year, almost, that he has been living here and regularly coming to talk — in the kitchen, in the late afternoon —, it bothers me to do it while he speaks. He hesitates, stumbling less because of gaps in his vocabulary or breaks in his syntax than because of his rough pronunciation. Then all of a sudden his sentences rush out, and now, on the cluttered table (newspapers, vegetables, crumbs), I can't find paper; I grab a newspaper scrap, or a torn envelope, a random pencil — to end up barely scribbling, sideways, on the sly, sheepish.

And I am loath to interrupt him. Still, shouldn't I repronounce his words, or send his sentences back to him, recomposed?

*

O. often interrupts himself, his face turned toward the ground.
If he suddenly raises his eyes, I get embarrassed to be caught looking at him too intently. And what would he think if he had access to sentences like these, which describe him?

With his index finger he scratches the wood-frame — rough varnish peeling off, pine fibers — of the table (the top is enameled metal: the style of a good thirty years ago).

Noises coming, then, through the windowpanes — changing with the hours or the seasons. Wind, small bell hanging from a corner of the kitchen's low roof… Or, coming through the half-open garden door, chickadee cries, needle-like… Or…

But what is it, emanating from his existence, near-mute for so long, as well as from mine, often verbose, that thickens above the table, between our faces? A double, redoubled, helplessness.

*

Sometimes, I drop the pencil, give up…
I cannot take notes anymore whenever, at sunset (he is about to leave: he never accepts to eat here, he'd rather go to a bread line on the street, or to a soup kitchen, or will do his own *petite cuisine*"), he starts speaking in outbursts.

Tomorrow, at the darkest moment before dawn, will certain words of his, beyond the breaches of sleep, reappear and press me to transform them into my own sentences… although, to be sure, mere sketches still?

*

"Come on, get going"… "…not a life," "not-my-a-life…": words exhausted with helplessness, blows from the hand or the arm or the voice, against what masses, surrounding them from all sides…

Those very words,
why did they have — at the moment (early May 2008) when I undertook to "set" (sour and dumb, that word) the notes I'd taken of our conversations for nearly a year —
to fly back in my face
    and

                                            at the risk of making me unable
                                to fulfill the promise I had made him months before,
                that of making — but for whom? — what he would say legible some day

NOTES

> ... without, it's true, his ever showing the slightest concern
> about this project
> except, just once, for a (perhaps ironic) remark
> on my endless delays — comparable (thought I, vaguely bitter)
> to the appointments he sometimes missed, his lapses or
> oversights?

stop me?

*

So, May 20, 2008: O. had just come home with a document from the Prefecture (where — mistakenly, in our judgment — he had gone unaccompanied): a residence permit (a "pass," he says) for **a month.**
Whereas, until then, he had been given three-month permits.

Why, I wondered, this reduction? What could be the reason for this sudden restriction concocted by the administration?
I went on to imagine (in a bout, as happens too often, of inefficient, even dangerous, panic) that the process officially begun a few months before (after more than two years without any kind of permit) would come to a halt... and then what... expulsion...?

But no, **three days later, O. received a summons for the signing of an "integration contract."**

Except that in this document (which I read to him, since he could not decipher it), he was being asked yet again — but this may have been due to the sheer automaticity of administrative forms or rituals — for a passport.

Where he was from, he explained to me one day (as he attempted to do with the administration), he had never had any papers. Only in the city did one have papers. In his village (one hundred and fifty kilometers from Nyala), there was no such thing. Identities didn't need to be written. An "old timer" would remember people, everyone and their relatives; and should that old timer falter, or die, another one was ready to take his place.

Today, however, he added (in the same harsh tone that comes to him whenever he notes the impossibility of knowing what became of his family after his escape — his mother, his sisters, alone, without a man), hadn't the old timer who would have remembered him disappeared — ended up displaced or dead, along, perhaps, with the whole village?

*

But first ... to begin ...
(whirlwinds of access — everything should be reopened simultaneously)

what "proves" that he is actually from Darfur?

the OFPRA,[15] then the appeals board — in 2005 — did not give credence to his explanations and assertions, during hearings whose interpreter seems not to have understood his Arabic very well, at least not his pronunciation ...
The (sketchy) grounds for denial incriminate the way he speaks, deemed "stereotypical." Was the idea to insinuate that the details on Darfur he tried to provide in response to suspicious questions could have been gathered by him outside of Darfur — in Chad, for example, among refugees (crowds, some camp's surroundings ...)?
(Or rather — grotesque avatar of "our" oratorical tradition and of "our values" — are the candidates for legalization, in order to "succeed" before these boards, expected to wield an art of persuasion that would also know how to mask itself elegantly?)

*

"See": it's often (soon after coming into the kitchen) **by this word that he begins,** sitting down in front of me (under the lamp ... music still playing in the next room), to tell his story, to try to explain ...

"See ... This is not-a-life" ...
Less life (less rights, less possibilities) than all others?
With all the others from Darfur who like him had found refuge on the banks of the Loire, he had been taken to a center to wait for his file to be reviewed. But he is the only one who hasn't been legalized. Seen as other, from now on, even by them. Falling through.

*

NOTES

"see…" — *to have fallen once more, no support left*

in the streets, so many voices,
and faces suddenly felt too expressive,

or alone by the river (ever liable, for those who survive on the islands, to
swell, brown-threatening)

when it rains, the concrete vault of an arch, under the railway bridge,

and always looking for food in the streets
and coming back to fall asleep on the ground

waking up to wash in the muddy water,
nothing to change into

"see"
… discouraging, the simplest self-care,
for someone crushed by fatigue and dampness, limb by limb,
into as many unliftable weights

stinky rubbing of skin or inflamed membranes
against themselves
mud and secretions dissolve or weld them
into the folds and seams of clothes

touching yourself makes you sick

*

when it was too cold,
buddies from the shelter would sometimes smuggle him into the kitchen where he could sleep for
a few hours, head on the table (at five in the morning, get out…)
and at dawn wait for the opening of the multimedia library, for example, where
("they're nice, nobody says anything")
he could doze for hours…

*

But first, his name is not "Ousmane."

It's he who, suddenly, on **April 23, 2008** (we have been talking for several months), asked me not to write his "real name" — the one that now appears on his papers.

What name should I give him in what I am writing, I asked? He suggested that of a friend: Ousmane.
Wouldn't that be a problem, or, who knows, even dangerous, for the friend in question?
That friend, he informs me, is dead.

Ousmane was killed in October 2003, in northern Darfur, near El Fashir, as he was trying to cross into Libya.
Nobody, says O., really knows what happened. The whole group with which Ousmane was traveling, in "a big truck," was killed. The killers were probably Janjaweed, who must have known those travelers were headed for Libya, and wanted "the people's money for their crossings" — and the truck.
Everybody died, O. says again.

But Ousmane's death, how was it known? He had an identity card (he who had lived in the city) that the police found.
The head of the village ("see, it's not exactly the mayor, but it's a bit like that") was alerted, and he himself announced Ousmane's death to the village, to the family: his father and mother, his wife, his two children.

"He was 35–36 when he died.
He had been my friend for almost two years.
He had gone to school, he was intelligent. He could have found work.
He had worked in Eastern Sudan, on the Red Sea coast, in a port. He got married there. Then he brought his wife all the way back to Western Sudan.
In the village, he lived close to my house. Not the same family, but the next one over. My grandfather knew his family."

*

"Come on"... how to finally move forward?

Should I reconstitute O.'s itinerary, and — at the cost of recomposing what he said to me (almost never speaking chronologically, but moving back and forth in time) — make the actual stages follow one another?

Or should the succession, here, reduce itself to that of the notes that I've been taking for months (with, often, a few hours or even a night's delay) from our conversations?

*

From what unquestionable starting point, or at least chronologically obvious one, should I have begun? from June–July 2007?

That was, in fact, a second beginning.
In a street downtown, by chance, one Saturday evening, a festival night (the music one, I think), Hélène was approached by someone whom at first she did not recognize but who — though hard to understand (mumbling voice, slowly looking for words amidst noises or bursting sounds from the street) — managed to remind her of a meeting two years earlier. He happened, luckily, to have a cell phone (gift or loan from friends) — whose number he gave her.

The next day, a Sunday then, I called. It's not he, but one of his friends — Hamid —, speaking French pretty well, who answered me. And we made a date, the two of them, Hélène and I, for the next day: a Monday.

*

But shouldn't I first go back to the very first encounter (of two years earlier) between us and O.?
And connect what I am writing here — or rather that which (in June 2008) I am setting from previous notes — with what was said in pages published over a year ago in *Po&sie*?

On the banks of the Loire, a Sunday afternoon, in 2004, alerted by *Le Monde*'s Orléans correspondent, we had met illegals living in little concrete shacks — probably abandoned working-class garden-sheds — amidst the brush.

And then we had, at their request, taken two of them to a hospital (in vain), then to a doctor on call.
Those two we had finally left in the streets of Orléans, not without hesitating, at sunset.

A few days later, we had learned that the Prefecture had all those people transported to a temporary shelter, some twenty or thirty kilometers from Orléans.
(As for the shacks, they were very quickly torn down, and the grounds, cleared of brush, had been given over to Sunday strollers.)

O. was one of the two we had accompanied to see the doctor. He was also, of course, among those whom the Prefecture had a few days later housed in the Center where, we thought, they would be able, as refugees from Darfur, to await their legalization.

So it's after a long break — a near forgetting on our side, and for O. the catastrophic denial by OFPRA — that the relationship with O. was given a second start.

*

Yesterday, July 16, 2007 — noted almost a year ago —, late afternoon, at the Lutétia (in front of the cathedral — great whitish 18th-century face, neither old nor young, and suddenly turning orange in the evening, facing west… illumination of the Loire's sky —, and not far from the synthetic slab blocks serving as bureaucratic annexes to the Prefecture),

fourth encounter with O.
(after three others, where, as a first priority, Hélène and I had read the documents he was carrying in a greenish, crumbling cardstock file, which only his friend Hamid, also from Darfur, who was there, had been able to translate, a little, for him.)

It was the first time that O. came alone. Hamid couldn't accompany him this time around (appointment with a social worker).

Hamid, who during our three previous meetings at the same Lutétia had acted as interpreter, is only twenty-two. O. is past thirty.
Hamid has finished high school, studied English, speaks French, even if, with a permanent half-smile, he speaks too softly, too fast.

O. is — at least that's what I thought I grasped then, though I would later learn that his past is more complicated — a farmer, he attended Koranic school only for a few years.

During our first two meetings, O. spoke to us only through Hamid.
But toward the end of the third meeting — **July 9, 2007** —, I found myself alone with him, and I noticed that he spoke — a strange kind of French, which he learned by listening to the youth on the Loire's islands, and which I had to reconstitute, on the fly…

It's at the end of that encounter (the third) in the café that I took O. (a few hundred meters from there, near the station) to Carrefour, to buy him a sleeping bag and a small tent (light, instantly put up) (a little room, he said).

*

What he began to tell me about his nights outside,
if, feeling my way along, I tried to relate something of it
once more,
it couldn't be without incorporating what I heard saw or re-imagined months later, following him on the banks of the Loire, that day in November 2007 when we returned to the place (an empty house squatted in for a few days in the middle of winter) where of course no traces of his could be found

but where he showed me others,
about the same, he said,
for him, in any case, all too recognizable,
strange-familiar
ephemeral bedding hollow, nests of dirty grass,
body moldings, debris:
the very little left behind, when moving on in the morning,
by those who must always take everything with them in the streets
(blankets, a few clothes, a minimum of food: nothing can stay
there — the city workers are instructed to take away or destroy everything)

and each evening reshape everything
into a minimal coil of self-care

*

and supposing it were a child of mine, adult, already old, who for some impossible reason would be met in this way, exhausted, eyes blank, in some strange (or too familiar) street?

(terror confounded with tenderness)

time has collapsed before him he never stops falling in a ditch full of black rotting leaves... (the stench of an absolute grief in which to let oneself sink)

"COME ON, LET'S GO," "you're not going to stay there like that"... (and... helplessness multiplies — he no longer wants anything — he is no longer reachable)

"PLEASE COME"... impossible to yank him away from this decomposition he now knows too well, has too often tasted... "COME, I'M BEGGING YOU" "COME ON..."

*

July 16 (first strictly one-to-one conversation), beneath the vaguely inquisitive gaze of the café owner (who recognizes us already), I asked O. about his life in Darfur, before the violence — perpetrated by whom, exactly? this question will run through his later remarks — began or, at any rate, became intolerable.

He worked the fields, he said, with his father.
(No, I later said to myself taking up again and confronting some of my notes, his father, at that time, was dead. And in later conversations it was his grandfather he would be talking about. Or rather he must first have said: "grandmother" because, as he will explain, he was referring to his mother's father.)

What they were growing, I have a hard time figuring out. With his hand, he shows me the height of the plants.
We raised sheep. He insisted on the lambs, on the fact that they could be sold. He spoke of the market, and I did not really grasp what seemed important... a vehicle...

Suddenly O. slips in — like a quick extra message, and adding that it's the first time he is saying this (*will I, in a moment, returning home, draw from those words some satisfaction, that of inspiring confidence... pinkish halo of emotion*) —
that he thought of dying.

He talks again of the islands in the Loire, differently from last time — of one in particular that he likes. Beautiful, for him? "Yes."
There, people come — young people, young couples — till late in the night, two, three in the morning... Friendly? "Yes, yes" — "I listen to them."

*

After our meeting on July 16, a room, a recently fixed-up studio (shower, toilet, kitchenette) that we rent became available on the third floor of our house (vast old building, going back at least two centuries).
We made the decision (which would remain in effect — dangerously abstract? — in all that would follow) to invite him to live there.

On July 23, from the Lutétia, where we met up again — with Hamid once more —, we cross the Loire and come home. I show him the place. He says very quickly, or rather (face lowered, tears — of humiliation? — welling up) he has Hamid say: "I can't pay" (while Hamid translates, he makes a helpless gesture with both hands), "not even for water or electricity."

Silence where, suddenly, in vital connections, is too deeply felt what is most banal.
Noises in the walls...
Soft trepidation of permanences-continuities, of connections maintained everywhere at great cost: drinking water coming up (on the banks, the city had cut it off...) or "wastewater" (sink, toilet) evacuating, electric cables (we see some, heavy and black, through this third-floor window).

"Can't" — "Of course."

Silence. Swifts calling, or, in the light flowing in horizontally from outside, the streak of a swallow, flying and diving under the gutter nearby...

*

"I was afraid" ... **"At the bottom of the big boat, I threw up, I was sweating, I thought I was going to die."**
Begin with sentences like these, heard weeks later?

A beginning in the middle of the Mediterranean (between Libya and France), *in medias res*...
Use pathos?
O. didn't know what seasickness was. **"If someone gave me a cigarette, it would fall from my mouth."** He laughs.

"I thought maybe someone had given me something with the food. I didn't dare eat anymore. I was scared they would give us something and then throw us in the sea."

"I thought I'd never see my family again, my mother, my sisters. I thought about my grandfather."

It was in May 2004, and the crossing took 8–9 days: 2 days on a little boat (for fishing) ("made of plastic" — is that really what he said?) and 7 days on the big boat.
On the little boat where he ended up, 7 people: 4 Sudanese, 2 Somalis, 1 from Burkina Faso (the only Francophone).
Then on to the big boat with other illegals — 40? 50?

On the big boat, of course, the illegals aren't all together. They are hidden in several places. In each of the cabins meant for the personnel's sleep, and designed for one or two, 7 pile up.

We're afraid. People yell things we don't understand. We're afraid that the police will come: everyone will go to prison then, even the people working on the boat.
No talking, no coughing, no sneezing.
(O. tries to retrace, to remember himself... He senses that I'm trying to get as close as I can to the feelings of that moment.)
"Him, he's afraid," "me, I'm afraid," "that's not a thing normal."
"They took your cell phone, your watch, your lighter, your papers if you have any, before you got in the small boat: 'you take nothing!'"

We eat once a day.

How does one manage... to pee and to... — I'm the one asking..., I'm a little embarrassed — what terms should I use... Our words are always reserved, discreet. Embarrassed, but not too much, he laughs: you pee through a little hole (a porthole?). And for... the rest... in a plastic bag... and then you throw that also through the hole.

Upon arriving in France, by way of another small boat, he had to slip on a "company" uniform.

After disembarking, around 9pm, we wait till three in the morning. We get a cup of coffee. A guy picks us up in a truck, takes us to the train station, pays for a ticket to Paris. (Another time, or rather several other times, O. explained to me the smugglers' complicated guarantee system.)

If I got it right, in the train for Paris, there are only two of them left.

*

In Paris, it's morning, we are right there on the sidewalk, we don't know anything.

We'd like a "small favor," a little help, some information. We speak, several times, to people passing by. We always choose someone who looks like an Arab, who must speak Arabic. But always he's suspicious, doesn't have the time, doesn't know.

Someone else is passing by, speaking through his cell phone: in Arabic. We try again, we ask him.
He stops.
He listens.

"& whether this is living?"

To *"To that which never ends"*

"No," says Ousmane: **"this is not-my-a-life."**
It's at least the second time I'm transcribing **these words** that Ousmane, a Darfuri who has been living with us three years, said sitting in the kitchen one day:
they will never, those words, **stop shivering**… (even if lately — May 2010 — I sometimes sense in him, whistling while he repaints a freshly plastered wall of the house in white — surges of happiness).

*

this handful of notes is taken from a moving mass that is and will remain in progress

(more than a sequence, these notes should form one or several spheres of pulsating possibilities)

*

For whom, and where, and when, is this … "not a life"?

You have to make **their life impossible**, one of the Prefecture officers said — while organizing indeed the icy and hateful impossibility of any support for migrants, destroying every inkling of an existence that would be livable for them.

*

"Auswandern" — **to emigrate** —: the title of a unique and (among his works) incomparable drawing by Klee, dated 1933.
A couple, made of cross-outs against white, of wrinkles in chalky air, of incisions in any possible common element.

*

Quick! *it's a tiny, dirty war.*

Would this be my war, the one I forever expected? Gather in a few sentences — if not lives, at least instants of what's "between" lives. **Condense**, *furiously… Let* **instants** *(raw flesh) of intersected lives tell themselves projectile-like…*
Targeting what?

*

After a step taken (a sworn affidavit made out at a notary's) to try and break out of the impasse where Ousmane's "papers" are still stuck in early 2010; we (Ousmane, three French nationals — the Sudanese "witnesses" hurried back to work) go get coffee at the "Quick" near the station, in the shopping center (where I return compulsively each day)… Heat (after the biting cold outside, the frozen snow, etc.), steam rising from clothing or bodies. My journalist pal unexpectedly speaks of long and intimate conversations with a Muslim friend — Afghan? I already forgot. "He explained to me," the journalist said, "that one shouldn't speak about one's mother." Is that so? Ousmane (*suddenly joyful — because, I assume, of the support we came together to give him —, talkative, in his French where he now has plenty of vocabulary, but which he pronounces poorly, due in particular to the fact that — because he doesn't picture written sentences? — he divides words the wrong way, doesn't notice articles, etc. — "l'équipe" (one of those he worked with in the suburbs, cutting down trees along the Loire, for example) becomes for him "les quipes," and so a new word, shorn of its first syllable,*[16] *is born in the singular, as also happens, to be sure, with other words in his mouth*) confirms: the same is true in his country. "You see," he says (at home he often says "you see" to me), **"a mother is like a god."**

Was I frightened at that moment?

*

The day after my mother's death (February 1996),
I tried, drowsy in front of the bay window
— blankets of snowdrop flowers discernible before sunrise
(*but how to articulate what becomes, in the night,*
of their white, their green, so naively raw — piercing like minuscule, very sharp nails?) —,
to "tell myself" (obscure folding back of the self on itself)
something.

Did I then simply try to "note"
the semi-silence of five, six in the morning?

Hissings or external-internal blows
propagating,
blood in the ears, echoes in the
walls, boiler rumbling behind the wall,
or, in dark-pink peel-envelopes of aural horizons,
cars, rolling wheels of big
trucks or of trains on a bridge on
the Loire, airplanes sometimes...

Suddenly: a brutal (dreamed in the frozen torpor?) ring
— call or injunction?

What trail of mental blood has slithered-beaded
scratching the plastery weather?

*Nothing but a whistling from the black-scaly nostrils of the dog
who, in the kitchen, on its blanket on the tiles, must have curled up, massive, and huddled trying
to shield itself from the harsh cold flowing in under the garden door or through the windows' cracks.*

*

Am I trying — too naively? crudely? — to capture at times and retain — here for example,
in a faint network of already gray sentences —
what the urge to live is made of?
This re-indeterminating burn that we slip to one another (from whom to whom? at which
exact moments?) like a thing that exists only insofar as it slides from hand to hand?

(No..., this already, a moment ago, in the three lines above, was *saying too much*.)

*

One 1995 Spring day, room at "Sainte-Cécile,"
where — torpid time —
my mother survives.

Sitting in the sole armchair (green moleskin) where, henceforth incapable
of walking, she stays for hours (till someone finally comes to get her up, to lift her),
seems asleep. Her lids
are not quite closed: I half-see
drowned eyes through the tiny slits.

I look vaguely through the rectangular window (metal frame).
Rayon curtains, the bland odor, so familiar,
of what delivers almost exactly what's expected
(except for the dust, or the tiredness of substances
and the collapsing of forms).

Turning toward her: "I'm going to leave," I say,
"I'm going to work"
(**Work?** bitter — as though in traces left by coal-blackened fingers on the paleness of the
past — is the history of that word… between us).

She half-opens her eyes: "Why?" she wheezes.
"Do you want me to stay? — Yes"
"Why?" I say to her in turn, too fast, almost meanly
(with the impulse to slip in, to no avail, a "What good will it do?"
or: "In two minutes you will have forgotten!").

And from her bewildered whisperings, I then heard emerge a single, weak, intelligible word:
"**Nobody.**"

*

Another day *a note from April 1991 which*
I came upon yesterday night Nov 21, 09, while randomly picking up and browsing through an old
notebook before trying to sleep,
my mother, not yet in a nursing
home (my father had left her here for a few
hours and we were bustling around forgetting her a little), I heard her

— making, on the dark-green back of the armchair, small
flutterings of the hands, then, suddenly, her index finger pointed —
mutter (among other crazy and dark, threatening sentences):
"and there are some who will die."

*

These notes... de-dramatize them (free them from the inevitable minuscule poses and stagings of the noting self)?

Or unwrap them continuously from their protections against what (through any momentary "object") they are speaking about...

And then let them subsist but harshly spread out: insects, smashed on what wall?

*

"& whether this is living?"
Virginia Woolf, *Diary*, Nov. 25, 1928

"[...] So the days pass, & I ask myself sometimes whether one is not hypnotised, as a child by a silver globe, by life; & whether this is living. It's very quick, bright, exciting. But superficial perhaps. I should like to take the globe in my hands and feel it quietly, round, smooth, heavy & so hold it, day after day. I will read Proust I think. I will go backwards & forwards."[17]

*

July 29, 2007 8:45 pm — Through the old bay window, meshings of branches, stems, leaves are visible: they are dripping with rain, more or less far off, and variously lit (with nuances of green-brown, of mauve or purple) by the dimming day.
This randomness of plants and of their respective growths (or that of my gaze, of my position) — everything suddenly is so right, furtively vibrating,
in tune.
It burns, in the tenderly acrid air (Perugino), **this arbitrary musicality**, always new:
it resides — more than it ever did for human beings, in "our" though, *nose against the window pane, this "we," in what I tell "myself," is choking me like bland cake*

NOTES

acosmism —
an incomprehensible
    surprise.

*

1949–1950? Some Sunday evening…:
Window panes painted blue (to block what had been *June '44* air bombings in the middle of the night)… long left as though blinded, dazzled by the evening light.
Scents — time-clouding — of colors, breath of silhouettes made of scarred cement, or black metal, rusted in spots.
Cut out, in the rush to get back home, against the orange sky,
a water tower, a gas storage tank…

Graffiti — appearing on what surface? — of a devouring, infantile seduction: the dazzle of war.

*

and velvety yellow: the irregularly rounded, even
lumpy flanks of a few quinces, on the tree still

… sensations (Nov '09), none of which is vital nor necessary, but which, through their happenstance, offer what it is awful to be (and especially by organized hatred) denied…

*

"an infinitely precious and sweet wonder"
(a marvel to be brought out by allusive description only?)
Leopardi, *Zibaldone* (8?), I wrote down this passage in a
notebook from '91–'92 thus (today, in 2009) at least
seventeen years ago, and, foolishly, without further identification…
"… Describing with just a few strokes, showing but very little of the object, [the ancients] allowed the imagination to wander among those vague, indeterminate childish ideas born from ignorance of the whole. And a rustic scene, for example, painted by an ancient poet

with just a few lines, without any horizon, so to speak, would evoke in the imagination that celestial, billowing excess of hazy, shining ideas, imbued with indefinable romance and with a strangeness, an infinitely precious and sweet wonder, similar to that which made the ecstasies of our childhood."[18]

*

Adherence to life: received — even if it takes on the air of a simple and minimal appearance of self-approval, even if it is only a negligible redoubling
like a speckled stone jutting out, brightly-solid, under running water
which must have taken shape long ago and has to recreate itself, if it can, throughout a whole existence.

This adherence produced itself and keeps nurturing itself **in the very rough certainty that one was** and perhaps still is *even while sleeping, cheek against some support* held in life and carried, through light, as if in the palm of a hand,
wished, yes — from where? by whom or what? —, to be alive.

*

From several women who, barely teenagers, were deported (Anne-Lise Stern?), I believe I have read or heard that they felt certain (with trust? with pain?) they had to **bring something back to their mothers: their lives.**

*

"Something white, infinitely white": the color of terror? of the death of all connection, of the most elementary trust?
I tell myself I don't have room here to transcribe a poem by Ritsos, which one cannot read without devastation: one of his detention-camp poems. He tells of the **loss**, seeping among the prisoners, **of the most elementary trust … And it is as if everything were paler**
The poem first related how one of them seemed to wish to speak:

> *[…] No one*
> *believes him anymore; looks at him anymore — let him say whatever he wants.*

But when the poem then comes to form-formulate the non-relationship, it is through the most precise invention, in images that mold themselves, with cruel accuracy, on impossibility ("**glass mask**"!)

> *Not that we were afraid of this frightened one — not at all. A higher*
> *window, from the fifth floor, cast a soft glow down on him;*
> *lit up his face as though he wore a glass mask.*
>
> And us
>
> *we then covered our faces with our hands as if to hide ourselves*
> *or as though to prop up a leaning wall. Between our fingers,*
> *bits of plaster, stones, dust, coppery coins were falling;*
> *we bent over and we picked them up; without kneeling before him.*

Then comes the "white": a horrible calm?

> *And in the mirror, facing, something white, infinitely white —*
> *an old bone comb in a glass of water,*
> *and the serene light of water in the glass, in the mirror, in the air.*[19]
>
> *Yaros, 05.24.68*

*

Ousmane tells me about his maternal grandfather (the one who, after his father's death at Nyala, had gathered the family in the country, the one also — other bits of stories in the kitchen — who spoke with his mother in a language that Ousmane did not understand, the one, finally, who died shortly after Ousmane's escape... *whence the dread of having left women alone exposed to... what?*)
and what emerges from his slow-moving words *time, thanks to linguistic difficulties, slipping inside his thoughts,* is an often silent presence — but which sometimes told of earlier decades, of journeys across Africa.

*

Ousmane, I asked him one day, **what is beautiful for you?**
(This was before he repainted here, almost meditating beforehand, with so much taste: nuances, several shades of white, and pale ochre...)

"It's when I've made something, in wood, in clay, that can remain in the house, and that we can see several times, each of us, my mother, my sisters…"

*

To go out into the garden — **in a May dawn** full of mist.
Familiar little utopia of **a Lilliputian focus-soon-to-become-writing: to ramify oneself** into everything known *in rivulets of half-sexual childish curiosity among the tender flesh of plants, shining, pearling…*
so as to better guide, through every link, fold, heap, cohorts of little black insects, identifiable but always surprising,
so as to insinuate words — to then… disappear
absorbed (as though it were going to close on itself, lip against lip, such that one might finally never have been)
by the real

*

From the door-sill of a house crudely lit within, someone
cries out

cries out to whom?

to a child leaving on a bike (headlight crooked on the fender *an ochre-pink halo is going to start skipping on the shiny gravel of the road as it unfolds* the chain's clinking already fused into the noise of a lashing black rain)

cries, with an angry voice:
"At least, come back alive!"

Perpetual dawn?

…the night hours just before daybreak, draw them out… and let them crackle into white fissures — possible notes pearling, then, micro-freedoms (that will evaporate)…

*

Rough drafts — but in what way impossible to *really* take up again?

*

There are no words, when the sun rises, in March, **for the evidence** of the fresh **sky** or **for its** most real **substance** (nearly flesh) — thus nowhere to be found

it's luck

or something irrefutable

between the staggered trees
in the red air

naked cherry trees (strips of bark have curled up during winter, droplets of orange sap) or, rising above them, at the far end, theatrical and powdered, the cedar's branches…

*

Pre-dawn notes: what harsh *in fact* in them?

to write them — "set" them — is to retrieve them as they never existed,
and yet as though already there,
exactly as they (virtual graffiti during sleep, or between lopsided moments and states of the day, or in the street, or while dealing with something else entirely, etc.)
preceded themselves.

*

Materials, on hold still, some of **these notes?**
to be "reworked" one day?

what gesture would be needed then, what quasi-transcendent drawdown (as in the vault-like fold of a heavy blue-brown fabric), or what turn of a suddenly free hand in some unreachable fourth dimension?

(here today, nothing glides on these rough-hewn sentences except — reducing them to what they are — a blade.)

*

And now, by straining to set themselves here, these notes (as if searching for each other, palpating one another with antenna-sentences) tend to connect: here **the temptation of narrativity**, there **an attempt at more continuous questioning**...

Are they renouncing their autonomy then, their multiple micro-freedoms?

*

But also: might certain notes — like these — be bound to free, to unlock and **trigger** a more biting and grinding **activity** (like that of chitinous, orangy-black mandibles in endlessly laboring insects)
liable to become that, almost unawares,
of future notes?

with their minute perpetual activity, these notes to come would attack

they would know how to directly take on the settings of real things

clasping on vital holds piercing through beliefs-consistencies
from which they would squeeze out vital-dreamed saps

*

It was often, year after year, under the effect and through the struggle of other attempts dedicated to specific "subjects" (with dog-like persistence *such as my recent — yet how many years old? — attempt on the power of stupidity*),
that some notes will have oozed out...

excess, then, Prussian blue,
beading sweat...

And yet those are the very ones that will have kept colluding with ordinary indolence; they never ceased to incorporate time without aim, time at its most vitally dull.

*

At dawn, but so late (because never before noted?) — like odors, whispers, or parasites of the immediate — **mumbling "political sensations" are returning...**

... constitutive, in the years just after the war (second world war), against the cheek,
was the breath-odor — warm — of a radio set:
bakelite and dust, it emanated from a little dwelling behind a greenish canvas rectangle (stretched near the small glass pane bearing the names of stations);
a tiny light bulb, orangy filaments, burned there

voices, perhaps of the micro-characters housed there, were twitching, moving...

twangy voices in the cheap kitchen we had then: they came from the depth of space as they come today from that of the past

arid, soon came the time of the Korean war, 1950–53 ("Time of the world: Korea," Vittorio Sereni wrote then),
it crept in like one odor too many among those kept within the family

*

... and Indochina? Algeria? enormous masses, orangy pressures inflections incurvations of the entire past

to have them come ... in what kind of after-the-fact attention,
to dilate them bloody earth-clouds

at last to rip them to shreds, furiously, in a corner, making up for the child who could not ...

*

ah! (8 o'clock, early March): what is it that just blinked a minute ago, outside?

in the black ramifyings, which seen from here against the pale dawn sky (through the old panes, warty in some places), appear as fine
as mesh

...what... a palpitation **was caught — the beat**, probably, of a (backlit) wing, wood pigeon or crow...

and everything felt, vibrating like a web, was
briefly certain

nothing "necessary"... but... if that
never happened
again... then... what
death?

*

The simple truth is that they are impossible to set, these notes: no sooner do they capture what they desire, however little, than they lose all stability.

*

For a lifetime: "perhaps-poetry"?

no name for that of course, long ago, during childhood, post-war years (coming home, in the evening, in the orangy gray street... white, gaping rubble)

impossible, in those days, to talk or to tell oneself anything about it...

and yet: **poetry as wrenching?**

a distant hope... to recognize at last?

to take hold
at certain moments (in the scents of grasses clinging to the bottoms of walls), by the sole weakness-strength of sensation
of what moving powers that
turning back against "me" — *against the burden that it proved impossible not to be for oneself*
would have wrenched me from my place
or would have seized back my own reality
— to rebuild it and
make me become substantially what would no longer be, in the end,
a "self" but mixed with unfettered breaths, bright spells, quivering alterities...

*

Nothing, in these notes, will have really set itself in motion if they don't palpably simultaneize themselves (in what flashes of evidence?)
with
what others must be feeling
— meaning me as well (the question coming back more vividly to me for having traveled "outside") —
of the desire or the hope, vague perhaps but lasting, to "account for oneself"...

What can I know, perceive, guess of it, in the street for instance? What else besides paltry ideas, crude representations (nothing supposedly, among "people," but resignation to their slow collapsing, or a vague decomposition of the "self"... — but no... maybe not...)?

*

Political, at least some of them — since the beginning — these sensations? Or will they not, rather, have been resistances or objections to any (effective or possible) politics?

Foaming with rage among the most familiar, often powerless, these sensations...: rebellious? "petty bourgeois"?
No, no... I am dumbly disfiguring ... how can I sketch out what shuns contact there, and flees?

*

Abrupt realism (upon waking) of ties or links and connections:

a shower in the night (jumble of wisteria branches vaguely lit up by the fanlight) (frost outside?):
the warm water in the noise of the water heater, its heat, I suddenly feel it as though subtracted from what?
and then, unexpectedly, the water, the gas, the electric wires, everything is recalled as what it is: pluggings, holds on forces, on realities prepared elsewhere, on time drawn off, a kind of sap circulating escaping and…

disgust, suddenly, from this multi-umbilical sensation
inside the steam?
dangerous, the sprawling dependency achieved in this way *everything will always be able — even willing — to turn itself off or run dry*

*

"What do we depend on to make us feel alive, or real? Where does our sense come from, when we have it, that our lives are worth living?"
Adam Phillips (quoting Winnicott: "If you show me a baby you certainly show me also someone caring for a baby, or at least a pram with someone's eyes and ears glued to it. One sees a 'nursing couple'.") [20]

Dependencies, yes, forever? Consubstantialities of lives… (Henry Moore: ties made real — in bronze).

*

To cast off, finally … what? To make oneself more than naked?

Hwang Ji-u: "When I take off my clothes in the bathroom, there is something else I would like to take off." [21]

*

A continuous and untearable attention-lining for everything that could happen...: might these notes be so many splintered traces of the search for a realization that one generally gives up on (settling for daydreams)?

The "mine" or the entirely other, vibrating from one minute to the next?...

A translucent alterity drawing itself out for everyone through the whole day, molding itself on events of all sorts, **glued like a tunic to the tiniest instants**, and consuming them as they come...

Intimate utopia... spouting, at times, irrepressibly, for each of us? — in the weariness of the street, on a train or in the course of compulsory chores...

the inevitable in everyone
and, simply, exposing itself in these notes?

*

Or: notes, right away, virtual at least, swiftly plugged to the cuts, the intersections of time

and above all drinking
between sleep/dream and
waking

: they must divert their life there
where the expectations or doubts of the day before, reopening themselves
(in the brusque gestures of getting dressed again..., struggling with the odor tubes or branchings that clothes are...),
can only,
vessels cut off in the air,
weep psychic substance

*

Swarms suddenly reappear, in dawn light, or under the kitchen neon, and teem (just when I thought I had set some sentences: these few notes)

micro-terror...
more than any others, the sentences of the "notes" should never make one forget those, half-formed, multiple, fleeting, contradictory, which came before them...

Wouldn't any unifying-crushing completion give these notes the flavor of a lie..., a smell of smashed insects?

*

Are they always being reborn, these notes
...sketches proliferating like vegetation dried from the start?

in order to elude any power of a whole taking shape and requiring each local outline to yield to the totality, to sacrifice itself or, at least, to let itself be precisely contained by whatever would measure its place...?

This instance of a "whole": would the work of art in Flaubert's "absolute" sense — and as "received" by Kafka — find itself tacitly confronted to social identity in the modern sense, to the nation state and (massively projected for example in Salammbô*) to its sacrificial monstrosity?*

(What can be felt of that in the constant evasions of these notes?)

*

And that other proliferation, of words in conversation?

Pig, I said when I saw myself (having broken away for an instant, almost against my will, from the conversation upstairs) in the dirty mirror above the café restroom sink, you are flushed pink from verbal arousal.

What got into me? why this volubility instantly belying everything I would have wanted to believe I cared about?

Does that arousal (heat on the cheeks) show up in my notes? *I asked myself, sickened, on the train, in the street, at night, crossing the Loire.*

*

"Above all I should have to be on my guard against those phrases which are chosen rather by the lips than by the mind, those humorous phrases such as we utter in conversation and continue at the end of a long conversation to address, facetiously, to ourselves although they merely fill our mind with lies — those, so to speak, purely physical remarks, which in the writer who stoops so low as to transcribe them, are accompanied always by, for instance, the little smile, the little grimace, which at every turn disfigures the spoken phrase of a Sainte-Beuve, whereas real books should be the offspring not of daylight and casual talk, but of darkness and silence."[22] (Proust, *In Search of Lost Time*)

*

The inner chatter: inevitable — or even quasi-corporeal, and bubbling, vital?

so… to discover oneself continuously in the process of secreting a flow of quasi-words? is this the necessary material for all that one can try to think/say? how could one join forces, making sentences, with this pattering production?

*

What, before any speech (or after it, swallowing it back),
*simmers and sloshes **"in the head" of everyone** right in the middle of the street*

what bits of sentences, anticipated, malformed, restarting, cooking…
all to suddenly make way for that which, irreversibly, happens to be said

*

… from a (self)mocking poem by Zbigniew Herbert: "**The inner voice**"…

(this kind of mythic existence of the inside… about which we know nothing until we speak and it makes itself heard by others or by the self as other,
this presence that is more real than anything, and yet constantly virtual…)

"[…] *it's hardly audible / and almost not articulated // even if you lean way in / you hear only syllables / stripped of meaning […] // sometimes even / I try to speak to it / — you know yesterday I refused / I've never done that / I'm not going to start that // — glou — glou*

// — so you think / I did the right thing // — gua — guo — gui // It's good we agree // — ma — a // and now take it easy / we'll talk again tomorrow / it is no use to me // I could forget about it […]" ²³

*

Accuracy: might it come only after some proliferation, vain at first or more or less ludicrous? Must it be called forth, and made painfully necessary, by sentences that are stifled-stifling at first… and in need of… healing?

*

When does it come at the right time, here (or when would it come, if it did), **the moment to set sentences: with a fierce listening gaze,** to strike the over-abundant

bend like a beak, poke around, rip to shreds…
lighten up with piercing voids…

… find the rhythm in a *second phase*?

*

As though induced by overly thick sketches (greenish soup),
it may — must? — suddenly happen that (animated by what forces?)
an intense spatialization
worms in and rages

… spacing, yes, breaths, tacit-tactile judgment, unfoldings freeing themselves abruptly, or some non-unifiable at-the-same-time, prevailing,

(aren't there then being created
— as though under the weight of falling/rising footsteps, tearing brown-mauve holes in the white —
places, possibilities to "count"…?)

*

… what, then, would be analogous to … "law" (in Lefort's sense)?

a breath-force spacing or lifting all the word positions in a sentence or a line of verse

analogous (no, something more: it is surely the same impulse) to the weights-positions of lives lived "in-between"?

each of us proving to be ourselves only through the passing of the self into whomever, indefinitely

*

"laws burnt in the lightning of stillness" [24] (Nelly Sachs)

*

To be recognized also, in these notes, possible materials (for a time that will only come dubiously?)…

piles of mental earth, heaps of confusion, construction sites abandoned in what wave of panic (flight…)
and left gaping in the rain
in the white air…?

*

At times, again and again, furiously, to hammer away at the already done, the too-completely-formed-formulated
— and to redecompose it in micro-entities, escaping, getting lost in the fog?

*

To return (sometimes traveling back years, sometimes a few days or a mere two or three hours) **to what, in general, I wrote, would that be to slide along my own corpse?**

Skin that is still alive against icy not-quite-dead skin… Cold bodily sweat in-between, in the half-life / half-death contact…

... in front of a barracks guardroom (in Lorraine),
in the middle of the night, in that police van I'd only managed to enter by crawling and groping,
it was all at once,
and with my own whole body,
that I discovered that the young soldier (twenty years old like me)
whom I'd just been told was hurt and waiting for aid
in fact was already cold

and then one had to ...

Alone, Khaled?

March 2015 – August 2015

"I don't want to be alone" Khaled said

those words, I will never stop hearing them again ... and the hushed, grainy, so very familiar voice
closer than close even today
— although

*

*not to be alone, but to be lost,
it's as if one's own pain and that of another
gave birth to a third heart*

Vladimir Holan, *En marche*[25]

*

only a start, these lines, *in the helplessness:*
a bit of too soon too late
nothing, here today, but a
"let it be said"

*

today?

*in the time — day after day, from hour to hour — when masses of migrants
are fleeing to "our place"
the unlivable reigning in "their place" (those hells in whose expansion
"we" will have
blindly or cynically
taken part)*

NOTES

news on **July 29, 2015,** France Musique 7 am ...
migrants trying to get through Calais to England

Khaled too, in 2006 I think, had made an attempt
— he admitted it to me only
belatedly and allusively
... out of shame? regret?

or, at random, from *Mediapart*: the day after the drowning on **Wednesday, August 5**
off the Libyan coast, the Italian coastguard announces 370 survivors ... the boat that was carrying at least 600 migrants capsized, then sank.

why bother to insert these two almost instantly outdated news items here, where hundreds and thousands of other images could-should pour in each day

visions available of rubber rafts of the Medusa deflating
(the other day at a Sudanese friend's in an Orléans suburb project in a short video on a cell phone handed to me
I heard an invisible helicopter whirring while an orange shape turned over on-in the sea, while heads could be seen: floating, disappearing)

(non) countings of vanished bodies

that's when our **"among ourselves,"
made of lives thinking of themselves as ordinary,
becomes septic,** *oedematous,
cyanosed*

*

*so "in" this computer will have waited, are still waiting — in vain? —
thousands of notes — quasi-instantaneous, factual, if possible, to the point of brutality —
for a **"With Khaled"***

*disparate and repetitive traces, gathered for eight years and which "should" be taken up again
shabby, dry gritty
quasi organic: dirty*

*

but wasn't it first
the actual things to be noted
that had endlessly amassed

bits of countless conversations
evidences that flashed for a minute
fears-angers laughter questions without answers
clarities and doubts

*

gather all of that in the coming months, raise it,
lift it up,
make it stand by itself
— forming what tombeau?

a Kleist-like vault *(the one he mentions in a letter to Wilhelmina):*
holding aloft only because all its stones want to fall

*

You, my friend! how I shivered from the chill of this
poem,
I was so afraid of words that I hedged again.
I would begin lines ... I tried hard to write
about something else,
in vain, and the night, this awful night lying in wait
commands me:
it's of him you have to speak!

Miklos Radnoti, *Fifth Eclogue* [26]

*

"not alone"

it was March 15, 2015 *a little before 11*
he had just come down from his room
he was, unlike his usual self, hesitant — gaze turned inward

he sat in the old green armchair
facing me
I tried as I so often did to make him laugh

but already probably
he could no longer hear me

he said that

*

those words, Khaled could not have had the strength to be afraid at the moment when he pronounced them…

but me, shouldn't I have been able on the spot (though it was a matter of minutes)
to guess
the catastrophe they were announcing?

he was there in the green armchair and I worried that he'd be cold (that spring morning was gray and freezing)

I led him back to his room (which in general — adjustable electric radiator — he overheated), I prepared herbal tea for him, handed him the cup

and

*

> *aren't I, talking about him, about this hesitant "us" that we were donning the rank and vain rags of mourning?*

*

> **I'd rather stop thinking if it's going to come out right away like this. There are thoughts, Julie, for which no ears should exist. It's not good, that they cry out at birth, like babies.**
>
> Büchner, *Danton's Death* [27]

*

*gathering — so as to form-formulate them —
a few handfuls of notes from the moments of Khaled's death*

*I can't avoid of course imagining for them
some possible reception
but right away it is
more insanely than ever
with
rage and revulsion*

**blood of rusting brambles
there it is again (from the depths of childhood)
the more than familiar
archaic taste**

**a delirium's
venom:**

**the sentences here
will
again start to twist**

**they are struggling to fulfill
the desire to be freed
from the desire to be welcomed**

*

Khaled Mahjoub Mansour, my Sudanese friend, on Sunday March 15 a little after 11am collapsed in front of me from a heart attack

for two hours they tried to get his heart to beat again

he stayed for almost three days in intensive care at La Source Hospital (south of Orléans) he died on March 18 2015, a little after 11pm

*

NOTES

on Saturday March 14, he'd returned from nearly two months in Sudan
a stay during which, for family reasons, he had to take an exhausting trip
that's what he began to talk about in our brief conversation (he was exhausted) that Saturday night
in a truck (to save the cost of a flight)
from Khartoum to Nyala

                                                         his home town, in Darfur

                         he had told me, in bits, about the markets where
                                             years earlier,
                 as a child he went to sell this or that with his father

                                        small vehicle…, small trips
                      and at noon, curled up in the shade under the stand,
                          tiny joy of a "little gift": a "little cookie"

an interminable journey cut by a long interruption (due to some vague skirmishes),
so three or four days, in the extreme heat… at times without water
etc.

                                                     *

Saturday, March 14, around 3pm, after weeks of absence (all too rare, his calls from a cell phone… *often from regions without service, he told me during one of our hasty connections*)

it was from France that he had finally called
he was at the Gare du Nord

"hello hello" — I'd heard (immediately recognizing his voice)
then a familiar laugh
then
"hello hello it's Mansour the jerk"

                                                 that was our password
                                  the cheapest of our ritualized jokes
                                           tasting of old shoes

"ducks and jerks"
two ducks from the Loire drifting along the bank
where two men were walking,
pacing their stride on them

we two were going
in search of places where K. had once slept
(some months through freezing nights after which dawn
brought at times, he told me, thoughts of suicide),

"two jerks watching two ducks,
two ducks watching two jerks"
wasn't it in January 2008 that I had said that to him, those idiotic words?

that find, stupid of course, self-realizing right here,
he had immediately adopted it with a sardonic laugh

*

vital, the laughter between us — or as though underneath us…
(what I used to say to make him laugh, wasn't I getting it from him?)

infra-what laughter? infra you-me

we laughed at the fact of being someone
at the need, for each of us together, to have
to be someone

*

duck or jerk…
and a coincidence:
I just came upon, end of July 2015,
the 'Resultant – Preface' of
The Spare Mug (in Flesh and Idea)
by **Sony Labou Tansi** [28]

What my God is that idea one should die with? This one perhaps: "The bourgeoisie is so dirty that communism becomes childish." Yet one has to choose, at all cost. And here is my choice: Neither dirty, nor child.

NOTES

And if I chose, understand that the fault is not mine, it's my century's. All those who will choose with me are "jerkists" of course, but they will have some peace. The peace of the jerk, different very fortunately from the peace of the duck. And then, they won't be such jerks after all, since they will have foreseen something for tomorrow, while communism only foresees one great day and the bourgeoisie its own fall.

SLT

*

of the need to be oneself, will I have wanted again and again to believe

from the time of high school
(gloomy years — 1956 or later: Hungary, Algeria)

lectures
— for handfuls of listeners in a tiny room in Orléans —

against the Algerian war,
or on South Africa — a documentary film shot under cover in the mines, with
suddenly the singing of
Miriam Makeba —

…or, heard in the near obscurity
— the glimmer of an obscure lecturer —
some pages of
Michaux, and the amazement
of finally feeling — "to act, here I come!" — the action, yes, real
(still so after returning to the streets, etc.)
of unfolding sentences

that poetry,
active-decomposing,
more immediately effective than any self-assignation,
could free?

and will such long gone instants have been
one of the conditions that enabled
my attention,
so late, toward the end of my life,
to the reality
— massive yet suspended —
of K.'s existence?

*

he wanted to return to die at your house said Samba my Senegalese friend
can I believe it?

such poor certainty-tears

*

so we will never have had it, that conversation I was waiting for …

not only the endless day-to-day one, so familiar, which had been ours for eight years, and which we would have naturally resumed that Sunday, March 15, before pursuing it in the days and weeks and months and years that should have followed

but yet another, supplementary one,
more deliberate naively studious

the one by way of which Khaled would have guided me through crucial places

as he had sometimes done by the Loire:
we were looking for places where he had slept on the banks of the Loire
under that railway bridge where one night two of his friends were run over

in the return
that I wanted to initiate

and with which I will have to wrestle in the coming months
but henceforth
"alone"

it will not be granted to me to resort to Khaled
(catching him in passing, in one of those moments when he was whistling through the house or the garden)

NOTES

I will not receive the help — and the vital difficulties — of words he would have added, or of his silences,
to reopen what I noted thus from so many shared minutes, so many words exchanged during eight years

*

two voices

like long ago in the wake
of my mother's delirium

two trembling equal unequal sources
is this what I must realize?

at the cost of irksome typographical
fumblings
(characters or font sizes, "letter types,"
"justifications")

*

if each of the two voices were to really come and write themselves
his being admittedly only the one I attribute to him
but my own only happening thanks to what it will have received from his

it would be by re-imagining the suspension created by the other one

*

voices, truly, caught in these lines?
they would crackle and jolt
never ceasing to differentiate themselves

they would have to inscribe here
in feverish variations

their emission point, or the direction from whence they came
or their distance (very far-up close)
or their many speeds

without it being possible however to recreate
the differences in accent
(of longstanding or recent inclusion in the French language)
or of course

the ultra-sensitive
material singularities
of voices
— of Khaled's

*

voices that will have to inscribe themselves within lines to be formed tomorrow
only by re-imposing — through what brutal actualization? —

the formless space-time of migrations
which would rush in between us, there, in the kitchen, when we spoke

handfuls of rain and sand storms of red hate
downpours of uncountable lives-deaths
in the kitchen riddling the talking and the listening with red

*

"home!" Khaled cried joyfully
when, a few months after his arrival in this house,
we were driving back from one "rama" or another
(one of those "ramas" — Brico, Casto, Confo —
which we called "shitty")
in the suburbs of Orléans

this vast ancient house
(which barely escaped — by about a hundred lucky meters —
the bombings of 1940 and 1944
...I had told him that story)
had for a good forty years
hosted for a few days or for months or years
a number of "foreigners"

he alone however
knew how to live it, feel it, differentiate within it:
walls and floors
volumes of distinct natures
odors-savors or noises

NOTES

*

home!

Nuruddin Farah, *Yesterday, Tomorrow, Voices from the Somali Diaspora*, 2000.²⁹

Beginning of the Foreword:

As a Somali, I was swept into the vortex of our nation's political crisis in early 1991, soon after the collapse of Mogadiscio. I was living close by, in Kampala, Uganda, where I was a professor of literature at Makerere University. I remember flying into Nairobi when I received an urgent phone call from my immediate family.

Further down, Farah contrasts the refugees of Mombasa (the poor) with those of Nairobi (rich and plundering)…

In Mombasa, the refugees dwelt on spectral memories, of grenades falling, and of uncollected corpses rotting at the city's roundabouts. Distraught, I understood the deeper meaning of a Somali wisdom in which a high value is placed on owning one's own home, as this affords a greater sense of privacy, of self-honour and of dignity. My father, my son, one of my younger sisters and a nephew, who were among the first to arrive in the coastal city, shared rooms with people whom they had not known before. I remember my sister alluding to 'one's home being one's protector, a custodian to one's secrets, a sentry at the gate to one's sense of self-pride. Having no home of one's own, and no country enjoying the luxury of peace: then perhaps one is a refugee.'"

*

the opacity in the house *restlessly moving in broad daylight*
where individuation, the having to be oneself, is swallowed back, chewed again, spit out again, every day-night of opaque restituting and re-wrenching from one same mass of can-live again feeding separate selves

how did it become substantial welcome-exposure to interruptions?

*

it is in this durably vital mass, "ordinary" for some lives
that a number of **irruptions**
became possible
(from Ivory Coast, the United States, from Iran, Cambodia, Japan, China, Korea, Sudan)

> *"irruptions"?*
> *I'm searching for words —*
> *in the news, from sociologists, specialists*
> *is a specific register needed?*
>
> ***refugees, intrusion, hotspots: the new lexicon of migrations***
> *August 10, 2015 | By Carine Fouteau (Mediapart):*
>
> *"These past few months, the words characterizing migratory phenomena seem to have been invested with new meanings. Relayed through the public space, they feed fears, produce exclusion and buttress the security approach privileged by European authorities."*

or rather
interruptions *(in the vital continuity of family life)…*
and intersections

or in the course of time
complex **inclusions**, *unexpected, softly twinkling*
overlappings *among existences*

*

and yet it was with Khaled alone — and this was partially through receiving it from him, from his way of being —
that the urge came to me and persisted (obstinate, ferocious even, day after day, for eight years)
to note down

*

from the beginning, almost always in the kitchen open to the garden,
I wished — and soon he wished —
to talk, obstinately

at the cost of many small misunderstandings (he spoke but very little French, we resorted to a little English as well — and to gestures, or, on a piece of paper, to drawings),
of jolts

on the other hand, after a few attempts,
I gave up on noting down on the spot, before his eyes, any of his words

I needed to be clearly (perceptibly for him as for me) free to absorb myself in listening

*

what is it then to take notes?
a decision .... not without violence? brutality?

to take notes as I was going to do, for eight years,
after listening to Khaled,
would I have found this impossible — forbidden even — to do for
my children?

to them, I told myself one day, I will have
(gaping responsibility-irresponsibility)
given — contributed to giving — **life**

Khaled, I would have liked to help him, on the side (and finally, in vain),
to have at last,
or once again,
*...***a life**

*

I'm copying here a passage that I had set (for publication in an issue of *Po&sie*) from our conversations, and where, at his request (for fear of what?), he was named Ousmane (or O.):

> **Jot down what O. says**, for the year, almost, that he has been living here and regularly coming to talk — in the kitchen, in the late afternoon —, it bothers me to do it while he speaks. He hesitates, stumbling less because of gaps in his vocabulary or breaks in his syntax than because of his rough pronunciation. Then all of a sudden his sentences rush out, and now, on the cluttered table (newspapers, vegetables, crumbs), I can't find paper; I grab a newspaper scrap, or a torn envelope, a random pencil — to end up barely scribbling, sideways, on the sly, sheepish.
>
> And I am loath to interrupt him. Still, shouldn't I repronounce his words, or send his sentences back to him, recomposed?

*

O. often interrupts himself, his face turned toward the ground.
If he suddenly raises his eyes, I get embarrassed to be caught looking at him too intently. And what would he think if he had access to sentences like these, which describe him?

With his index finger he scratches the wood-frame — rough varnish peeling off, pine fibers — of the table (the top is enameled metal: the style of a good thirty years ago).

Noises coming, then, through the windowpanes — changing with the hours or the seasons. Wind, small bell hanging from a corner of the kitchen's low roof... Or, coming through the half-open garden door, chickadee cries, needle-like... Or...

But what is it, emanating from his existence, near-mute for so long, as well as from mine, often verbose, that thickens above the table, between our faces? A double, redoubled, helplessness.

*

... so: never take notes on the spot...

to have first been simply free to give one's attention without ulterior motive or calculation, without knowing what return you will get from this gift (just for the generosity — the intrinsic happiness — of the attention)

no (re)forming sentences until the next morning to give myself the time to "understand" what I will have heard?

take the time, rather, so that
all that was heard the evening before be bathed in sleep
or rather be restituted by dreams
to the shifting muds of belonging,
to the archaic jaws of ferocious dependencies

*

will I, dawn after dawn, have *reformulated* K.'s words?
inevitably, though less and less, over time, with his French getting stronger...

but also it was crucial to try to recapture, at the same time as the words and the listening, their own element, the pale reality, in the kitchen, of the between...

*

NOTES

> *reconstituting,* before daylight, Khaled's words of the previous evening seemed to me at times like *translating* a poem...
>
> the thing already said by another
> return it to the state
> of a cloud of lines, of crackling possibles,
> a stormy swarm
> decomposing-recomposing in the air
> in the between of lives and voices
> before redepositing itself fresh, burning
> on the page, or the screen

*

Khaled slid off the sofa where he was sitting, he collapsed on the floor right when I was trying to catch him in my arms

March 15 at 11

his head, eyes rolled back, was heavy in my hand; I felt his saliva leaking out

I left him for a few seconds — to shout in the stairwell (toward our friends, Jinjia, Aya, toward Hélène)

I returned to that collapsed body, lifting it up again, and crying

(and then very quickly the firemen, abrupt at first: "Who are you to him?," then the EMS, a Sunday morning, a doctor, who happened to be black, suddenly speaking, for his part, with caution and kindness: "it's very bad…" "the heart")

(he died after three days of treatment by a team of doctors who were completely attentive to him, to that body, which only artificial reflexes still animated — and at the same time, moreover, to us, setting time aside for us, dazed as we were, or for the Sudanese friends, for Youssef who took on the task of telephoning his mother, in Khartoum)

*

at this time (early August 2015) it's been a little more than eight years
since we came up, with his friend Hamid, who translated, to this studio — in our house
to which he would soon have all the keys
and while opening it for him
I told (had someone tell) him that he could live there from then on

he answered, through Hamid: I can't pay the water, can't pay the electricity

I said: of course
my eyes were stinging — and I saw his shining with tears

years later, he will tell me: "I was afraid not to say the right words"

*

> *And so, I didn't respond to your call, I didn't*
> *knock at your door ... but you, you, did you call me,*
> *really? ... and you would have opened the door for me, really?*
> *And everyone can say: I had no other path, and there*
> *I met whomever I could! ...*

De Signoribus, *The Round of the Lay Brothers: 1999–2004*.[30]

*

De Signoribus poetry

furtive evidence of referenced gestures immediately vanished
in the darkness

one will have felt their precision ... things and events were there for sure, within reach ...
and right away: suspension, evasion ...

will the poem have given up loading itself with news, with referential, documentary
explicitations?

it's rather that they instantly burnt it
all that is left are gestures retracting filaments
(and minuscule echoes of cries that glow and char)

*

NOTES

of course, Khaled knew that I was "taking notes"

once, he heard me read some of those notes, during a "gathering" at Maison de la Poésie, one Saturday afternoon...
(he was in Paris then
I had not suggested that he come, we had seen each other a moment before in a café on rue Beaubourg,
and it was upon leaving the reading that I discovered he had attended it)

you take my words, he had said, following our return, in Orléans,
(slowly like always, searching for his words),
you put in your words
you find the right words

*

did I believe want to believe for a second on this August 10, 2015 at 10:16 am that those creakings in the hallway were his footsteps and that he would arrive surreptitiously, ironically... pretending to surprise me in front of the computer... and then burst out laughing?

*

suddenly, at times, he would show up
in this room while I was
striving
to rework the notes of the previous day's conversation

burning to recreate
for his sentences or mine
(the very ones which, the evening before, had not stopped smashing
against invisible obstacles)

some vital element
in which they would no longer have to stop breathing

gills of free-moving sentences sensing the bloody nets that await

*

CLAUDE MOUCHARD

there would never be any "because it was him, because it was me"

we obviously did not choose each other

**only the brutality of the real (first: the catastrophe in Darfur, then Libya, then ...) will have landed him
in this house**
in July 2007

his bereft life whacked
as though by the slap of a wave against our protected lives

on and between our continuous lives his interrupted life

**and yet the one who (emerging from the monstrous anonymization of migrants)
lived here — was, "at our place,"**

he

*

we? family, home ...

whatever had been, over the years, the troubling moments (reciprocal doubts, debts, or costs, vital cruelties)

**a minimum of coherence, of continuity,
a core of consistency**

**such was the condition
to live**, to believe in, or rather dare **to realize**
— on our part
or on his
this life "with K."

NOTES

I felt him
over the course of weeks, months, years
become certain
that he could always count on us,
on the house

*

consistency, of course,
continuity, yes

but — and contradictorily? —
without giving up on shedding
the opaque self-caring of lives that want to be
or believe themselves to be
ordinary

or, by some impossible means,
without adding too much to the ever returning lie
— in its obtuse promises to itself —
of the "good life"

the one whose dubious certainties
I will have tried for years
to unfold, obliquely

without ever consenting to the devouring version (destroyer of possibles)
of coherence

without (perchance) being part of the viciousness of so many lives eager to consider themselves
"at home"

those who live their "every day" and their adhesion to themselves
only at the cost of denying the unexpected surgings
born within and of the obscurity of their very "intimacy"

those who project their own internal ruptures
(the sharpened edges that irresistibly take shape within them, between them, by them)
in order to change them into "outwards" violence and cruelty
against supposedly total others

*

it's for Khaled first, and it was nearly for him alone,

after Ibrahim-Kim-Pedram-Farzam-Laura
or, very differently for sure, but not without interactions,
Linda
or
Masatsugu, Jinjia, Aya, Méï …

(this enumeration limps and wounds:
— so many singularities!
and, for the last four, ties with Khaled)

and almost from his arrival here,
that the obvious imposed itself, imperative, blinding: I had to take notes

was it because he came from Darfur, where he had fled genocidal violence?

the kind to which, for years,
like a good many other intellectuals in recent decades,
I had learned to pay
special attention
— ethico-political? even poetico-political: in order to realize? —
but which itself had to — ought to keep being
subjected to a critical concern
(wasn't it already the "truth fever" conceptualized by Catherine Coquio?)

others however — Kim (the Khmers rouges), Pedram, Farzam (Iran, the Iran-Iraq war), Laura (Angola) — had fled extreme violence —

what specific change occurred with the arrival of Khaled in my double desire to not only listen, but strive daily to form-formulate?

*

until then (without thinking of it) I had
partitioned

it had been necessary for me to maintain
between two areas of existence
— that of presences-irruptions (or of the multiform availability and inventiveness they
required: for listening, or any number of life concerns)
and, quite close, quite different
that of my "own" attempts (to read-write, naturally, etc.)

I had worked on the condition of possibility for everything else:
a strict **separation**... never thought through,
simply incarnated in this very house, its volumes or internal times
I had obscurely obstinately maintained

an impermeability

*

*in the most
receptive spot
rises the wall that built
itself, and did so in such a way
that it could not otherwise*

Vladimir Holan, "The wall that built itself" [31]

*

**Yet Khaled too
partitioned**

in the three days between Khaled's collapse at our house and his death at the hospital,
and then in the weeks following, and today still,
Sudanese people, coming from Orléans or Paris or other cities — Lyon —,
have shown their care
and their desire for closeness

I had met a number of them, if not all,
at Khaled's, in his studio
but it was always briefly
— out of discretion (for which Khaled sometimes, humorously, reproached me: "you never
stay..."),

      but also, as one of his friends, Youssef, explained to me, because Khaled was clearly determined
                    (at least at certain moments and about certain points)
                  not to let an excessive influx impose itself in our house

                         … a few weeks after Khaled's death,
Jinjia, our Chinese friend (from the first floor of the house), as we were coming back from Paris together and
                             conversing in a night train,
                  picks up the term "partition" that I just used:
                         to partition, he suggests
                   — to maintain distinct zones of existence —
         was necessary for K., for the precarious "balance" of his living-surviving

and so, as I belatedly learned to understand,
when we spoke, it was he, there — and not all of him

for, even if it was just to talk in the kitchen
(and aware that I was going to take notes),
he had to maintain gaps within the ties themselves…

some non-crossings
without brutality,
with delicateness, humor

but in order not to make impossible… what? in his life… his relationships and ties?

        or sometimes, as if despite himself, he maintained portions of solitude
            between himself and us between us and the (Sudanese) others
                  between himself and the Sudanese

                         blades of emptiness
                        cold-blowing breaths?

             *

for me at least the partitioning
imperceptibly stopped happening

the impermeability between regions of life
in the family-like cohabitation with Khaled

could only as in a smile
give way

a mental wall no longer had any reason to be
consenting to its own uselessness, it had collapsed
blowing nothing but sweetness

an internal wall of the heart
cooked day after day by care

browned purple and crumbly

must have broken down unnoticed:

dissolved
in the limpid shade of affection for Khaled

vanished

ENDNOTES

1. La Chaîne Info: a television news channel.
2. Jérôme Valluy, "La nouvelle Europe politique des camps d'exilés: genèse d'une source élitaire de phobie et de répression des étrangers," *Cultures & Conflits*, n° 57 (spring 2005) 13–69 (see https://conflits.revues.org/1726).
3. Caroline Moorhead, *Human Cargo: A Journey Among Refugees* (London: Vintage Books, 2006) 1–2. Quoted French translation is from *Cargaison humaine*, tr. from the English by Marie-France Girod (Paris: Latitudes, Albin Michel, 2006) 3–4.
4. Varlam Shalamov. Quoted translation is from "La Quarantaine" in *Les Récits de Kolyma, Quai de l'enfer*, tr. from the Russian by Catherine Fournier (Paris: LGF, « Le Livre de Poche », 1990) 124.
5. Judith Soussan, *Les SDF africains en France: représentations de soi et sentiment d'étrangeté* (Paris, CEAN-Karthala, 2002) 96.
6. *Les SDF africains en France*, 113.
7. John Rawls, *Political Liberalism* (New York: Columbia University Press, 1993) 41. Quoted French translation is from *Libéralisme politique*, tr. Catherine Audard (Paris: PUF, 2006).
8. Claude Lefort, "La pensée politique devant les droits de l'homme," *Europa. Revue d'études interdisciplinaires* (Montréal: 1980). Reprinted in C. Lefort, *Le temps présent* (Paris: Belin, 2007) 405–421.
9. The source is in fact Jérôme Valluy's aforementioned article, "La nouvelle Europe politique…" (see note 2).
10. Union pour la Démocratie Française, center-right party.
11. Direction Départementale des Affaires Sanitaires et Sociales: department-level administration in charge of social assistance and public health (abolished in 2010).
12. Department store chain, selling electronics, music, and books.
13. Colloquial term for people of North-African immigrant descent born in France or other European countries.
14. Ingeborg Bachmann. Quoted French translation is from *Poèmes*, tr. François-René Daillie (Paris: Actes Sud, 1989).
15. Office français de protection des réfugiés et apatrides: a government agency protecting refugees and nationless people.
16. *L'équipe* means "the team," so *les quipes* assumes a word "quipe" (here put in the plural), which does not exist.

17. Virginia Woolf, *The Diary of Virginia Woolf*, v. III, 1923–1928 (London: Hogarth Press, 1977). Quoted French translation is from *Journal d'un écrivain*, tr. from the English by Germaine Beaumont (Paris: Éditions 10/18, 1977) 222–223.

18. Giacomo Leopardi, *Zibaldone*. Quoted French translation is from *Zibaldone*, tr. from the Italian by Bertrand Schefer (Paris: Allia, 2003).

19. Yannis Ritsos, *Yaros*. Quoted French translation is from *Pierres Répétitions Grilles*, tr. from the Greek by Pascal Neveu (Paris: Ypsilon Editeur, 2009).

20. Adam Phillips, *Winnicott* (Cambridge: Harvard University Press, 1989) 5.

21. Hwang Ji-u. Quoted French translation is from *De l'hiver-de l'arbre au printemps-de-l'arbre: cent poèmes*, tr. from the Korean by Kim Bona (Bordeaux: William Blake & Co., 2006).

22. Marcel Proust, *À la recherche du temps perdu*, t. IV: *Le Temps retrouvé* (Paris: Gallimard, 1989) 476. Quoted English translation is from *In Search of Lost Time*, v. VI: *Time Regained*, tr. Terence Kilmartin et al. (New York: Random House, 1999) 302.

23. Zbigniew Herbert. Quoted French translation is from *Zbigniew Herbert, Le Labyrinthe au bord de la mer* (Paris: Le Bruit du temps, 2011).

24. Nelly Sachs. Quoted French translation from *Eli, Lettres, Enigmes en feu*, tr. from the German by Martine Broda, Hans Hartje, Claude Mouchard (Paris: Belin 1989) 275.

25. Vladimir Holan, *Forward*. Quoted French translation from *En marche*, tr. from the Czech by Xavier Galmiche: www.espritsnomades.com/sitelitterature/holan/holanvladimir.html

26. Miklos Radnoti, *The Fifth Eclogue*. Quoted French translation from *Marche forcée*, tr. from the Hungarian by Jean-Luc Moreau (Paris: Phébus, 2000).

27. Georg Büchner, *Danton's Death*. Quoted French translation from *La mort de Danton*, tr. from the German by Arthur Adamov, in *Georg Büchner, Théâtre complet* (Paris: L'Arche, 1970).

28. Sony Labou Tansi, *La Chair et l'Idée* (Besançon: Les Solitaires Intempestifs, 2015) 45.

29. Nurrudin Farah. *Yesterday, Tomorrow: Voices from the Somali Diaspora* (London: Cassell, 2000). Quoted French translation from *Hier, Demain. Voix et témoignages de la diaspora somalienne*, tr. from the English by Guillaume Cingal (La Madeleine-De-Nonancourt: Le Serpent à Plumes, 2001) vii.

30. Eugenio De Signoribus, *Ronde des convers: 1999–2004*, bilingual edition, tr. from the Italian by Martin Rueff (Paris: Verdier 2007) 23.

31. Vladimir Holan. Quoted French translation from "Le mur qui se bâtit lui-même," in *L'Abîme de l'abîme*, tr. from the Czech by Patrick Ourednik. www.espritsnomades.com/sitelitterature/holan/holanvladimir.html

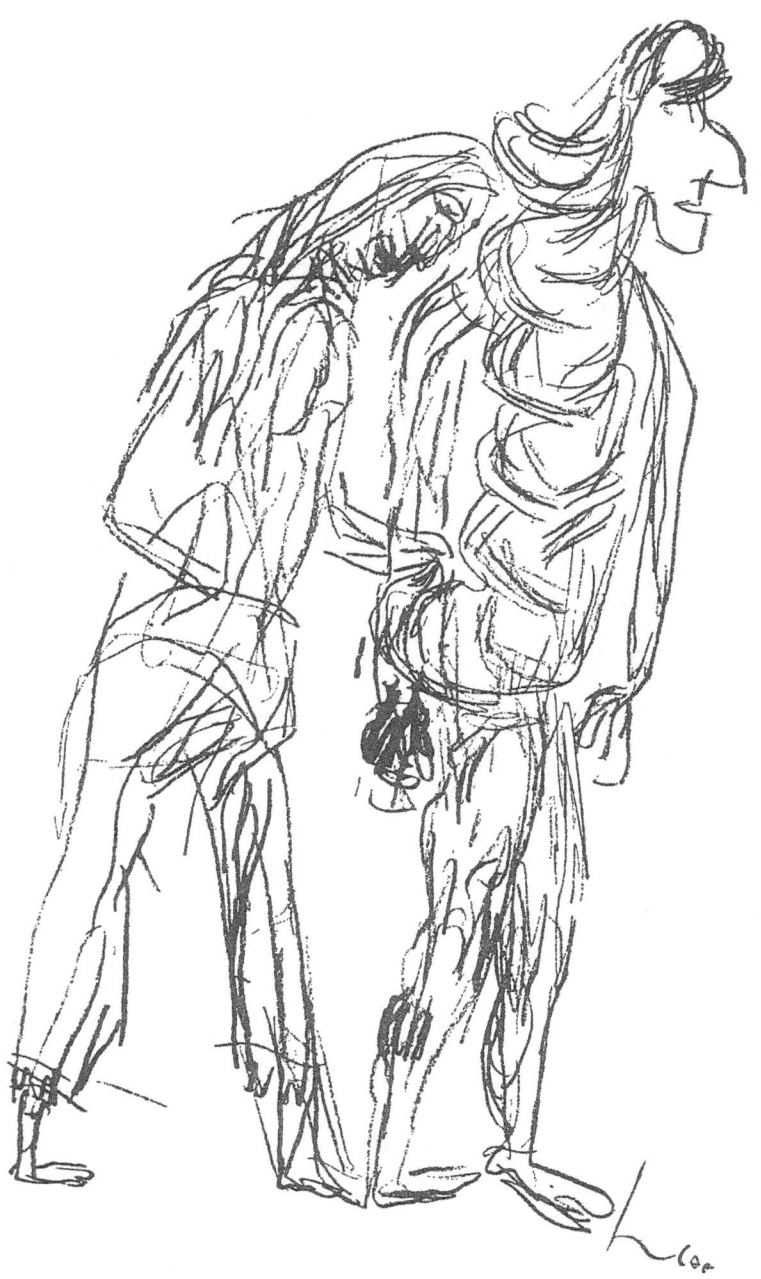

Auswandern (Emigrating), 1933, Paul Klee

Enchevêtrée

ELLE BUTE. Sa lèvre intérieure s'alourdit.
C'est la vieille méfiance qui s'est ravivée, mais d'un doute, je crois, tout nouveau.
Des parcelles de cendres flottent, sous les poutres, le toit énorme.

───────────────────────────────

Faire de ces instants une chose à raconter ? Je l'ai voulu (conversations…)
juste après — pour m'arrêter aussitôt.

───────────────────────────────

Son doute éblouit. « VOUS… », dit-elle,
debout dans l'embrasure de la porte de la pièce.
Elle tend son maigre index droit qui tremble…

Cheveux gris métalliques tordus dans la lumière, rudes, gros —
chacun pourrait être compté.
Voudrait-elle rester figée ?

Derrière elle la pièce voisine est, presque horizontalement, illuminée. Afflue, à travers la baie vitrée, le soleil d'un soir de début mars — répandu pâle et froid sur les champs où subsistent des chaumes de l'année précédente, des restes desséchés de tiges de maïs.

───────────────────────────────

Sent-elle autrement, maintenant, l'air ? Que voit-elle, dans les minutes, fibriller ou granuler ?
L'espace va-t-il cesser de lui être traversable ?

Le présent, ici écrit : grossier.
Il tente, souffle court, d'engrener ces phrases (leur durée) sur… ou dans… ce qui eut lieu alors

(ou dans ce qu'il faudrait ne pas laisser, simplement, avoir eu lieu — si du moins ne doit pas rester bloqué là-bas ce qu'elle essaya, donc, IN EXTREMIS*.)*

―――――――――――――――――――――
―――――――――――――――――――――

La radio, à peine audible dans l'une des chambres. Porte mi-ouverte ; courant d'air.

Arrive (disons) : à travers le creux probablement brumeux que forment les prés proches, un cri — de vache, de poule — ou, de plus loin, portés par des sautes de vent, des cisaillements minuscules et incessants de centaines de pintades sous des tôles.

Elle a les mains fermées, les tenant à hauteur de la poitrine,
silhouette où dansent d'autres silhouettes.

Elle dépend entièrement, maintenant, soupçonneuse, exposée, du geste que je vais faire ;
la prendre par le coude,
la conduire lentement jusqu'au fauteuil rouge sali face à la cheminée récente en briques.

Est-ce du doute qui respire par elle

ou, très vieux, un désir de croire qui
    cherche à re-brûler
        — pour passer hors, s'évanouir en rougeoyant…

―――――――――――――――――――――
―――――――――――――――――――――

Il n'y a, à l'évidence, plus rien de familier pour elle. Tout se retourne vers elle, contre elle, l'arrête.

Tout se fait brut
    (grisâtre ? ou follement coloré ? *Ni moi ni elle n'accédons à ce qu'elle sent*)

et lui colle au visage,
        rampe sur ses cornées qui larmoient.

Du moins, dans cette pièce trop vaste, et trop provisoire
        (charpente nue d'étable :
    de molles masses de poussière accrochées aux échardes du bois se
        déforment continûment,
            du blanc palpite dans l'air)

où j'ai eu tort de la faire venir et où il faut maintenant la guider doucement, est-il une chose qu'elle découvre avec joie :
le feu.
Elle en parle soudain, d'une voix à peine distincte.

Bruit dans la cheminée :
du bois brûlé s'effondre ou c'est du métal qui grince en se dilatant.

Des flammes — dont elle se met à commenter (à petites exclamations émiettées, exaltées, presque imperceptibles)
        les sursauts (vent s'engouffrant) qui brusquement
           l'illuminent, la chauffent —
elle,
    assise comme elle est maintenant,
ne se lasserait pas
    (pressent-elle en même temps ce qui déjà
        s'est insinué, obscur, avide,
            et enveloppe et confond ses pensées ?)

Mais tout à coup, ce qu'elle remarque plus vivement encore, c'est,
    revenue des champs et des haies (buissons sans feuilles, longues
    herbes couchées jaunies par l'hiver, tiges de menthe qui rampent —
    et trouées de mulots ou de couleuvres)

sa chienne noire
qui, courte et frétillante, lui pousse la main du museau.

« CHIENNE » ? C'est trop dire.
Car justement, dans ses marmottements qui maintenant se bousculent, volubiles,
elle ne lui donne pas ce nom.

Serait-ce qu'elle ne dispose plus du mot ? Il semble plutôt *(en ai-je alors été sûr ?)* qu'elle
(l'évitait)
L'ÉVITE

CE PETIT CORPS TIÈDE ET NOIR, agité, se dandinant dru,
brillant d'une laide *(pour moi ?)* condensation

appartient évidemment au plus que connu, au « fait pour »,
      à tout ce qui, *pavillons et jardins de banlieue,*
      rues dessinées,
      framboisiers et rosiers, pyracanthas,
      se croit ultra-prévisible,
      voudrait se voir *(arêtes de crépi, lignes pauvres)*
      transi d'évidence,
mais il en jaillit, là,
      dit... dans la grange (le vide) par cette vieille bouche,

    à dire pour
    réaliser en éclat la banalité
    chair qui n'est formée que dans l'air,
    par ses souffles et ses gestes,

    et mange — de sa puissance de mélange et simplification —
    le nom que je pourrais encore vouloir lui donner...

…fluctuation,
(salive qui brûle)…
tous les mots seraient-ils à cet instant
potentiellement touchés, doucement affaiblis ?

———————————————————

N'a-t-elle pas, dans ce qu'elle ne nommera plus jamais,
…je le sens moins en regardant
la chienne
(même si, blottie contre elle,
elle est l'exact résultat de ce qu'elle a voulu)

qu'en essayant, suivant les indications courtes de
ses chuchotements, ses ébauches de gestes

de discerner ou de condenser
(en même temps qu'elle, mais autrement)
juste devant son visage ou tout près de ses mains
dans le soir bleuâtre

une tache, instable

glissé et logé (dissimulé ?) depuis des années,
un peu de ses plus vieilles
   (contractées, là-bas, sous la première guerre mondiale)

ALLIANCES OU RÉPULSIONS

ANIMALES

— celles qui, héritées, séculaires,
étaient menacées — dans ce qu'était devenue une vie comme la sienne, de ne pouvoir passer plus loin

et de devoir rester
inchangeables et cruellement affamées,
au fond de son enfance — là où débouchait du temps très lent,

là où resteraient pour toujours en attente odeurs et respirations enfantines-animales

    contacts
        flanc contre flanc ou cuisse,
            peau ou jupe de fillette
                contre laines et pelages ras
                    au crépuscule, moutons et chiens

        rapprochés sur le bord escarpé du plateau,
        et, émanant des écroulements de pierre figés
        ouverts juste avant la nuit

        (*je l'avais, enfant, perçue en elle bien avant de*
                savoir ce que c'était),

        la terreur — dents de fer.

———————————————

« ELLE », dit-elle, sollicitée encore par le museau humide.
Ou, soudain : « ÇA ».
Moins que mots
    émis palpitants dans l'air de plus en plus froid
        où flottent des poussières ou des parcelles de cendres
        (*soleil très bas, feu, avancées d'ombre*)

———————————————

« Elle »…
Ai-je suggéré : « la chienne ? »

…« Elle », répète-t-elle, agacée, « ça ».
Elle a entendu le nom que j'ai dit, mais elle m'ignore.

Ramassée dans ce vide,
il lui faut de minute en minute,

se soucier de cette petite… quoi ? …présence ? la soutenir…
où ?
Foyer « elle » plus que chair-chienne halo pulsatile
elle l'entretient de mi-mots qu'elle mâchonne (bribes verbales et sensations)
en pâte ensalivée

sous ses gencives faibles mais obstinées
doutes et certitudes s'égalisent en continuité laiteuse vitale
pour « elle » pour
« ça ».

_____

Elle chuchote : « elle », « ça », ELLE ELLE MMM
        elle la nourrit de sa continuité de gorge et salive suc

      LA PETITE PRÉSENCE ça oui elle DANS HORS

…*est-ce que je sens alors graviter*
des pôles d'identités se concrétisant bleus lunaires
              dans le soir précoce de mars
ses souffles (chch, mm) se font-ils suspens de positions et de rapports

selon elle — « elle »
POUR LE LIEN À ÇA… ?

_____

ENCHEVÊTRÉE

Pâle, la nuit, dans le vasistas au-dessus de nous.
Elle murmure, elle chantonne.

———————————————

Me fait-elle (sans le vouloir, bien sûr) entrer une seconde dans le comme si des contes

comme lorsque dans le mesquin appartement au premier
   le temps était condensé par la guerre, la neige,

      et que à hauteur des feuillages de platanes tout, entre les murs, en dépit de l'angoisse, jouait ?

———————————————

…de la métamorphose bat…

même si elle ne parle presque plus, et si elle
      semble ne pouvoir guère, elle, maintenant
         que souffler — n'est-ce pas
            rythmiquement, avec de très courts effets ?
…et se pourrait-il que selon son murmure la tenue de tout… change et que tout écart s'emplisse
   — de quelle substance soyeuse, de quelle boue de réalisation-mutabilité ?

———————————————

Elle somnole, éclairée par le feu qui baisse.
La chienne s'est endormie, enroulée sur ses genoux.
Tout s'est-il allégé ?

_____
_____
_____
_____

Cris — d'oiseaux de nuit. PATTES sur le toit dansent soudain.

Elle se réveille. Elle n'a peut-être dormi qu'un quart d'heure.

Comme son visage, alourdi, est fiévreux
et amère, sa bouche !
        La chienne s'étire.

Voici
    (c'est là que je voulais — croyais vouloir ? — en venir…)

qu'elle
me raconte
    (à moi ?
    non : c'en fut alors fini, une fois pour toutes,
    des récits à moi ou à quiconque adressés)

passionnément,
quoiqu'à voix à peine audible

        pour l'écouter continûment
            (elle qui parle non à moi mais au vide),
      est-ce de me sentir effaçable que j'ai besoin ?

      je fixe, pendant le long de l'un des murs en plâtre, une
          ampoule, sa lueur froide (pression…)

qu'elle l'a vue, « ELLE », donc,
non plus bondissante, mais…

…comme elle était triste ! se plaint-elle…

je l'ai vue, dit-elle
        (pas à moi, dans le vide),
se coucher, oui,
non,
SE LAISSER TOMBER sur le seuil de l'école.

Couchée, « elle »
sur la pierre
corps étalé — ayant subi, « elle », « ça », brutalement humiliée,
quel refus ? rejet ? —

pantelante, douloureuse, sifflant
à l'entrée de la cour,
    sur, donc, probablement,
        un rugueux bout de calcaire
            (bribe de falaise grise orangée) (mousses, herbes)…

Oui oui
    c'est là   marmotte-t-elle
        (elle martèle à mi-voix, doigts tressautant sur la chienne
         d'opaques formules de colère)

c'est de là
    (flamboiements sur les parois en brique)
    la voici qui s'indigne dans l'obscurité

qu'« elle »
regardait.

Assise (vieux fauteuil), c'est en regardant le feu
qu'elle
       …voit ? croit voir ?
sent et dit *(l'un par l'autre)*,

qu'elle forme dans le vide ce qu'« elle »
       (en quel temps ?)
voyait
       du seuil où elle était couchée, tête sur la pierre,
       gémissante,
       au fond de la cour,

ce qui pour « elle » (comme jadis pour elle ?) pouvait,
là-bas, à travers les arbres,

brûler briller PROMETTRE…

―――

…lumière de l'unique salle de classe —

j'essaie de discerner (comprendre-sentir)
— autant que par ses bribes de phrases,
  selon les éclipses, ses souffles (*oh, ah, mmm*) (émerveillement, indignation, tristesse)
jetés dans le noir —

ce que c'est (*maintenant ?*), ce que c'était (*jadis ?*) ou pourrait être

    POUR « ELLE » ? ELLE ?

ENCHEVÊTRÉE

de croire la voir…

concentrée sous les tilleuls,
infuser, si sûre,
brûlante ?

MAIS QU'Y AVAIT-IL AUSSI dans cette lumière,
de faux,
de nécessairement méchant ?

> *Rayonnant ambiguë*
> *elle, la lumière, attendait, elle devait attendre*
>   *(décoction jaune limpide d'ailes d'insectes, de*
>   *graines noires)*
>   *pleine de sensations antérieures*
>   *à rejoindre*
>   *sécheresse de la page sous le flanc de la main*
>   *ou, s'écrasant contre le bois peint ou la vitre,*
>   *les craies de couleur odorantes,*
>   *éblouissantes, cristallines*
>
>   *(ou même — sur une jupe en laine*
>   *couleur terre — immobile,*
>   *feuille sèche, regard, une mante*
>   *religieuse)*

qu'elle offrait — ou
   refusait.

———————————————————————

A cette promesse brillant là-bas, reçue d'où, ayant subsisté où, autre, (trop forte ?)
   (promesse… tu sais bien… : « Jude » !)

c'est maintenant enfin,
dans la nuit de la grange

qu'elle — si faible, égarée, incapable de se relever du fauteuil —
objecte-produit
ce mixte corps hors noms,
« elle »
cette réelle-irréelle chair cruciale.

───────────────────────────

ON L'A REPOUSSÉE
        crie-t-elle à voix basse, se redressant un peu, avec peine,
        bouche qui tremble, pommettes enflammées
oui, on a refermé sur elle la porte que les enfants venaient de passer
        excités (cela, elle ne l'a pas dit),
        après avoir dévalé du plateau par les chemins alentour,
        riant, se bousculant,

Comme elle avait couru, pourtant !
        crie-t-elle encore (doucement).

Et voici qu'elle restait là. Seule à rester là.

Elle, ça, la chienne ? elle, elle. Mais oui : ça.

───────────────────────────

Elle pleure, visage plissé qu'éclaire le feu.

Ses mains se lèvent au-dessus de la chienne endormie,

    avancent dans le vide,
    osseuses (hématomes),

    tremblantes, véhémentes,
    accusatrices.

Qu'est-ce qu'elle cherche encore ?

Elle bourdonne de ce refus auquel elle dit avoir assisté,
                qu'elle voit, là…

Et, se soulevant un peu, comme dans une vague de protestation, de souci…, de dépit,

« on devrait… », souffle-t-elle.

―――――――――――――――――――――
―――――――――――――――――――――

MAINTENANT il lui faut rassembler SA COLÈRE
— pour la dernière fois —

abstraite,
haletant grise dans l'air
contre quoi ?

Elle aurait besoin d'amasser les objets de sa colère
    mille objets contre lesquels je sais qu'elle ragea
    mais —
        énormes (14, 39, ciels enflammés, exode,
          Indochine, Algérie)
        ou apparemment dérisoires
        (à la campagne, en ville ou en banlieue, sur les
            routes) —
    dont elle ne voulait rien savoir que sa rage,

qu'elle aura toujours cru devoir
ne jamais commencer à comprendre
(pour n'y avoir pas la moindre part)…

pour sentir une dernière fois, d'un seul coup, rayonner
d'eux, à travers eux entassé

vers elle, contre « elle »

ce qui
lui apparut toujours
comme disposant, s'abattant,
    sacrifiant… stupidement ? ignominieusement ?

    — décisions plus ou moins souveraines
    (mourir pour ou ne vivre que selon)

    mais devenues (pour elle ? pour tant !)
    grotesques, nues, sanglantes

_____

    …je doute dans l'obscurité, à ma façon, je me défie…
    tisons, froid…

_____

    pour « elle », pour « ça »,
    (s'élançant, avec les enfants,
        odeurs d'herbe, bruissements de
           feuillages)

    c'est la promesse même — lumière, là-bas,
        entre les branches noires, au fond
    de la cour —

*qui s'était soudain défigurée
dardant du refus*

*ou qu'elle découvrait, avec « elle »,
        apparentée
à tout ce que toujours elle avait haï*

*ou plutôt : elle venait de la forcer, cette
lumière, cette promesse à se révéler
arbitraire*

*aujourd'hui… là…
pour « elle », pour « ça »,
pour ce qu'elle formait
sur-le-champ,
— mixte, humaine-animale,
        grotesque…—
à cette fin que ce qui venait dans
cette lumière-promesse
se manifeste
sans plus de justification
dans un pur flottement
(qu'elle disait selon la plus courte colère
et selon le mélange,
remâchant les distinctions et positions,
les noms…
mi-mots défaits, écumant, donc, mousse
— rage et doute —
quasi visible dans la nuit
scintillant sanglante)*

ON NE LEUR APPREND RIEN,
      détache-t-elle soudain d'une voix étonnament claire, à CES —

elle se crispe comme sous un coup,
à la différenciation elle s'est recognée

à…

on…   *(elle s'est remise à pleurer, faiblement,*
        jeunes vieilles larmes jouant à glisser,
           à briller avec le feu)

    (elle remarmonne un instant)

on ne veut pas *(reprend-elle fermement)*

il faut *(voici exactement ce qu'elle a dit)*…, on veut qu'elle reste toujours COMME ELLE EST.
Et pourtant
      a-t-elle repris, vite
          (avant qu'on ne l'entende ? non,
            avant — si ç'avait été encore possible —
              de s'entendre elle-même)
je suis sûre qu'elle pourrait…
ÇA — oui —
    tels furent, oui, ses mots
APPRENDRAIT

ÇA SAURAIT…

    Et puis souffle interrompu, toux et froissements :

        chaumes ou plumes poussent dans la gorge
           la voix s'y perd.

ENCHEVÊTRÉE

C'était fini —
elle avait plus qu'assez tâtonné…

VOUS…, *répéta-t-elle — au vide.*

Elle se tut (à si peu de choses près)
   pour des mois, pour quelques années, pour toujours.

LE SILENCE.
   Elle s'endormit enfin profondément — bouche s'ouvrant

La nuit.
Mais sous l'effet de cette flambée
      — une ou deux heures durant —
je fus encore,
            indécis, perdant contours,
la possibilité, la substance
d'autres points de confusion
         dans l'air de la grange,
taches ou zones d'indistinction (minimes, bourbeuses) revenues de loin, ou naissant là — mêlant
de l'humain, de l'animal, ou des générations, ou des choses, des feuillages, des herbes

n'importe…

Elle ne parla presque plus, jamais.

Avait-il fallu que fût sur le point de s'araser son pouvoir ou désir de dire

pour que cette zone de mélange redevînt
    — pour elle et (dans une certaine mesure) au-delà d'elle, ou à côté, de proche en proche —

plus réelle que tout ?

―――――――――――――――――――――――――

…et fumée… et voiles gris se mouvant…

―――――――――――――――――――――――――
―――――――――――――――――――――――――

FUT-ELLE DÈS LORS QUELQU'UN ? Comment ?

L'accent subsista

résistant à la quasi-perte de la parole il passa dans la mélopée que peu à peu elle se contenta de chuchoter

il ne cessa pas d'être la vieille différence au plus près
capable de se diluer
sans disparaître
nuée orangée ou brun noix fleurs
lal lalie
se perdant dans l'eau des sons

(Y AVAIT-IL ENCORE QUELQU'UN ?)
(dans la coque des os, sous l'oreille, la tempe)

— et comme jamais — enfin —
légère !

Papiers !

Pour Jean, pour Daniel

Canaries... Des barques sortent de la nuit sous des projecteurs. Puis, sur un quai, des corps titubent, soutenus par des hommes gantés de plastique blanc. Est-il resté des morts au fond des barques ? (Des cadavres seront probablement rejetés sur la côte. On en verra des images.)
C'était sur *France 2*, le lundi **2 septembre 2006**. À une heure tardive, il est vrai. Mais qui n'a pu voir des choses comme ça ? Photos, dans *Le Monde*, dans *Libération*, etc. Et internet.

Tout le monde a vu, chacun sait, etc. **À quoi bon**, *ici, faire des phrases ?*
(Ou en recopier ?)

En plein soleil (un peu plus tard, dans le même reportage de *France 2*), deux hommes, des adolescents, plutôt, marchent sur le quai. Ils ont été débarqués là quelques semaines auparavant. Ils ont pu (nous apprend la voix off) rester sur place, engagés comme interprètes. L'un d'eux dit : « si j'avais su, je serais resté dans mon Afrique, là-bas, il y avait toujours quelqu'un... »

4 octobre 2006 : vu par hasard sur LCI, un habitant des Canaries (dont la voix nous dit qu'il s'occupe de clandestins — en tant que psychologue ? je n'ai capté qu'au vol, j'ai oublié, déjà) avance (*mais son soupçon lui-même aurait-il à être suspecté ?*) que les autorités du pays tablent sur ces afflux de clandestins pour obtenir des aides européennes.
Il insinue aussi que ces sans papiers seraient exploités par les entreprises de bâtiments — en plein boom touristique aux Canaries (au long de ces plages où — comme le montrent d'autres images — des baigneurs parfois découvrent des corps rejetés par la mer).

Échelles de bouts de bois... de n'importe quoi, grappins absurdes, contre, sur, des barbelés...
Fin septembre 2005, ou début octobre, ç'avait été (comme on a dit) l'« assaut » (quel mot !) aux bords de **Ceuta** et **Melilla,** enclaves espagnoles en terre africaine.

Libération du 27 mars 2006 :
« Les grillages de Ceuta ou les barrages électroniques des Canaries ou d'ailleurs ne décourageront pas tous ceux pour qui la galère d'un clandestin en Europe vaut mieux que de croupir dans un village sans espoir au Sahel ou la banlieue oubliée d'une mégapole africaine. »

Que peuvent-elles,
ces bribes (informations, souvenirs d'informations) ramassées ici
(et tout de suite décrochées des présents… : dans le vide)
susciter de mieux que nos habituels soupirs (en éteignant la télé) :
« ça ne devrait pas » avoir lieu…, ça « n'aurait pas dû… » ?

Les clandestins, s'ils ne sont que les résidus, dans « notre » présent,
d'un avenir où tout serait réglé et chacun à sa place,
*comment **pourrions-« nous » réellement y***
***penser** ?*

La question des clandestins serait-elle d'emblée
périmée ?

Et encore, et indéfiniment :
« Il y a d'abord les yeux, hagards, apeurés, qui errent sans trouver où s'accrocher dans le tourbillon d'images nouvelles. Il y a les bras qui se tendent pour avoir à boire, encore et encore, et étancher l'inextinguible soif… »
Benoît Hopquin, Los Christianos, *Le Monde* du 14 octobre 2006

Ces citations, ou d'autres (combien d'autres possibles !),
les transporter ici, les donner à recevoir (par les phrases frustes d'ici),
*est-ce sentir-tester **l'attention** qu'elles*
*auront supposée ou auront tenté — **en quel « nous »** — de susciter*

(à la suite, bien sûr, de celle sur laquelle n'ont pu que compter
les « yeux », les « bras qui se tendent »)… ?

«Nos» bords, «nos» frontières...
Et plus loin, ailleurs — là où on «externalise» le traitement des migrants clandestins ?

«Les projets dits d'externalisation de l'asile sont apparus fin 2002 dans les débats européens, pour désigner des politiques tendant à délocaliser dans des camps placés hors de l'Union Européenne les procédures d'examen des demandes d'asile ainsi que l'accueil des demandeurs d'asile et des réfugiés. Elaborés par des gouvernements européens en collaboration avec le Haut-Commissariat aux Réfugiés de l'ONU (HCR) et la Commission européenne, ces projets visent à créer des «zones de protection spéciale» dans certaines régions du monde (Afrique centrale, Moyen Orient...) afin d'y concentrer les réfugiés et d'éviter ainsi leur migration vers les pays européens.»

Régler le problème des migrants là où celui des droits de l'homme ne se posera pas... ?

«En amenant les États voisins puis, plus largement, les Etats «partenaires» (notamment dans les programmes de coopération, aide au développement et action humanitaire) à faire le travail de rétention, d'enfermement et d'expulsion des migrants en transit, s'opère une externalisation non plus de l'asile mais de la répression et de l'enfermement des migrants.»

Du Caire — 30 décembre 2005 (envoyé spécial du *Monde*) :
«C'est comme si un ouragan avait frappé la place Moustafa-Mahmoud, à deux pas du centre-ville du Caire, dans le quartier chic et tranquille de Mohandessin. L'évacuation forcée par la police égyptienne de 1500 réfugiés soudanais, la nuit du 30 décembre, s'est soldée par au moins 23 morts [10 enfants, 7 femmes et 6 hommes, est-il précisé plus loin – et *«tous anonymes»* est-il ajouté] et par un nombre inconnu de blessés parmi les réfugiés, et a transformé la place en un champ dévasté.»

Au Caire — où se cachent-ils, les «garçons perdus d'Afrique» ?
«... à l'origine, la formule désignait les jeunes Soudanais séparés de leur famille en fuyant la guerre civile dans les années 1990.» (Caroline Moorehead, *Human Cargo*).
«Il y a beaucoup de garçons perdus au Caire. À vrai dire, ce ne sont plus aujourd'hui des garçons, mais des jeunes hommes originaires de Sierra Leone, du Liberia, d'Éthiopie, d'Érythrée, du Soudan, de Guinée, de Côte d'Ivoire, du Rwanda et du Burundi...»
«Au cours des dix dernières années, ils sont arrivés par différents circuits, à pied, par le ferry, par avion, par le train, en camion, à dos de chameau ou à cheval...»
«...persuadés que, malgré les horreurs, la vie valait encore la peine d'être vécue, que l'Égypte allait leur ouvrir les portes d'un avenir pour lequel leur passé de victimes de la barbarie des guerres civiles et des conflits modernes leur servirait de passeport.»

« NOTRE » BORD, que devient-il, et que deviennent
aujourd'hui
NOTRE « DANS », NOTRE « ENTRE NOUS »

…tout autres qu'il y a quelques années ou décennies ?

*Des barques glissant hors de la nuit sous des projecteurs… Ce fut
celles de Vietnamiens ou de Cambodgiens…
Eux, on (= « nous » ?) les cherchait,
on leur tendait la main…*

3 janvier 1980 : c'est la date du « journal intime d'un chrétien rescapé » que « Kim »
(qui, peu avant l'invasion de Phnom Penh par les Khmers rouges,
avait achevé ses « études dentaires »),
ayant fui le Cambodge, et enfin réfugié au camp de Chanthabury (Thaïlande),
a écrit à la main, en français et en anglais
pour tenter d'obtenir d'être accueilli aux Etats-Unis ou en France
(journal qu'il a finalement laissé ici, « à la maison » — là où (octobre 2006)
j'en recopie, telles quelles, deux ou trois bribes) :

« [...] Malgré la fièvre, la faim et la fatigue,
j'ai réussi à m'aventurer seul pendant deux nuits et 3 jours
à travers plaine inondée du mois de novembre et forêts
dans des zones frontalières strictement contrôlées de la province de Battambang. »
[Mais la faim, explique-t-il, le contraint à s'approcher d'un village, où il est aussitôt arrêté…]
« Je sais qu'une mort atroce, cruelle va m'attendre dans peu de temps. »
« [...] je suis surveillé et suivi de près, dans une pagode abandonnée,
avec ma section de petits soldats-guérilleros habillés en noir.
Dans le pays, ce chef est réputé par ses actes de génocide.
Quelqu'un le croisant en chemin, n'ose pas voir sa face,
se courbe l'échine et lui cède le pas avec respect.
À mon exception, aucun prisonnier qui lui a été livré n'échappe à la mort.
Dans l'enceinte de la pagode, j'ai vu des fosses,
fraîchement comblées de terre souillée de sang humain [...] »

…Kim, sorti d'un camp en Thaïlande, avait été pour quelques jours hébergé
dans un centre d'accueil du sud-ouest de la France

> avant d'être conduit à Orléans,
> **ici** (nous avions donné notre adresse en réponse à un appel paru dans Libération),
> **où il arriva**, boitant lourdement,
> décharné (nuque d'oisillon assommé nu sur un trottoir),
> *pour*... enfin
> **manger**
> (mêlant dans la poêle sur le gaz, en un bain d'huile crépitant,
> des œufs, des sardines, du beurre),
> et pour — à la faveur de ces quelques mois, ici, donc, avec nous —
> devenir (non sans amertume, non sans moments accablés d'impuissance)
> aide-soignant pour des vieux... des
> corps blêmes bleuis fripés.

...nous

me dis-je — où ? à la maison ? dans quels endroits de la ville ? en quels instants de nos vies ?

que devenons-« nous » —, mois après mois, sous l'impact de ce qui nous est jeté par les journaux ou la télé, ou par la présence (massive furtive) de ceux qui (à travers déserts, mers et montagnes, barbelés, menaces et contrôles)
arrivent – « nous » arrivent ?

En quoi nous métamorphosons-nous dans chacun des cas où nous prétendons « nous »
> (notre « entre nous » — dont l'évidence n'est évidemment qu'image aussitôt décollée,
> écaillée —,
> notre prétendue « manière de vivre »,
> nos droits — à nous réservés ? marques de quelle élection ?)

protéger de l'irruption
(ou si nous tentons encore de l'ignorer) ?

> ***Comme d'une pression de paume trop fraîche*** (opaque-éblouissante) sur les yeux,
> **quand le « nous »**, dans les rues, dans les lieux différenciés de la ville,
> (ou dans l'« entre » tourbillonnant remordu en l'air)
>
> ***se rabat-il sur mon attention***
> — celle de qui, non-migrant,
> **sédentaire**
> *aura toute une vie piétiné les mêmes lieux* —

pour m'écarquiller, me réécraser
en deçà *de moi*
— de cet être-soi dont, comme quiconque, j'aurai été chargé —
et me défaire dans l'air en taches fluentes de libre réceptivité
sans retour sur elles-mêmes… ?

Le « **DANS** », le « **NOUS** » : **en sentir** crûment, dans l'odeur des rues, sur le pont, à la maison (dans l'entrée, le couloir, les différences d'air entre les pièces),
le goût ferreux, les déchirements, la violence ?

L'« **ENTRE** » chaud rougeâtre, *réexhalé partout des corps en mouvement, des visages tels qu'ils s'y projettent*,
comment l'effectuer tel qu'il se révèle (mais en se redérobant aussitôt, redoutable) **aux instants où** les effets de **son bord** (de la détermination de celui-ci — ou celle des accès ménagés — par le pouvoir) s'y font sentir
ou dans les lieux-instants
où ce bord même **passe au milieu**
c'est-à-dire
    toujours, sans doute, en s'abouchant, noir fluide, aux divisions internes du « dans »,
        à ses équivoques et renversements,
    mais spécialement, violemment, insolublement, **aujourd'hui, par les « clandestins ».**

Dans une « **VILLE SÉCURITAIRE** » comme Orléans

là où j'essaie
(chez moi, oui, protégé, certes : dedans familial ancien… portes, vitres,
murs (qui de toujours, à vrai dire [depuis la guerre — mondiale], parurent irrigués de nuit) —
*de **fixer ces phrases***
*sans, peut-être, **arrêter***

> *leur remâchement au cœur de l'élément même*
> *du « dans »*

— terrain, depuis plusieurs années, d'expérimentation du sarkozysme —

> *par exemple dans les rues descendant vers la Loire qui, anciennes, étroites,*
> *ont été repavées blanchies :*
> *fabrication d'un « nous » de moutons féroces*
> *pour lequel il a fallu lessiver, sur les murs, la vie du temps*
> *(effaçant les précieuses couches noires-rouillées à déchiffrer : balzaciennes)*
> *et réaliser, irréversiblement, l'idéal idiot où*
> *la moindre pierre est travestie en (comme dirait, à peu près, Deguy) elle-même*

comment, là même où les regards sont guidés, ne pas sentir ses propres sensations longées
par des sillages
les arrivées furtives de ceux que des passeurs auront ici (de préférence à Paris ?) abandonnés,
dans les rues, en pleine nuit…

> ***Tchétchènes,*** *il y a deux ou trois ans, signalés*
> *par des membres d'une de ces associations*
> *qui seules essaient de veiller*
> *(ressource que Sarkozy a entrepris de détruire)*
> *en train d'errer dans l'obscurité sous la pluie de novembre…*
> *H. y va… :*
> *pourparlers sur-le-champ — puis, dans les jours et mois qui suivront :*
> *médiations, résistances, transactions avec les institutions, etc.*

> ***Et qui étaient-ils, ceux entrevus***
> *(par H. et moi, passant par hasard en voiture)*
> *un soir glacial,* ***au centre de la ville,***
> *entre musée et cathédrale,*
> *et à qui (depuis une camionnette) la Croix-Rouge*
> *elle-même empêtrée (instrumentalisée ?) dans quelles négociations*
> *avec les « autorités » (la préfecture, masse blanchâtre non loin de là ?) —*
> *distribuait de la soupe… ?*

« Il faut qu'ils souffrent » aurait dit, il y a deux ou trois ans, un fonctionnaire
de la préfecture.
« De peur qu'ils s'habituent. » « De peur qu'ils en attirent d'autres... »

Au bord de la Loire (rive sud, à un ou deux kilomètres peut-être à l'est de la ville), à l'écart de la route,

dans une de ces zones confuses où semble régner une vacance des contrôles (mais trop éloigné, cet endroit-ci, de la ville pour que s'y passent, comme dans d'autres comparables, des trafics, des affaires, entre autres, sexuelles)

saules, osiers, masses *qui, sous le vent, dans le courant, se renversent
soudain*
si clairs *(unis alors au ciel),*
hautes broussailles,
bandes de sables variables,
odorante boue de Loire nuancée et merveilleusement fine
(comme celle puisée au creux d'un sabot
dans quel conte d'Andersen ?)
et oiseaux, rongeurs de toute taille

rives qu'on apercevait, à la fin des **années quarante**
(pont cassé, effondré : blocs obliques, tiges de métal),
depuis de longues barques noires

ou bien, à vélo, quelques années plus tard,
dans la mi-obscurité où les chemins se perdaient,
sentir (sol déroulé sous le halo des phares) le réel
grésiller en possibles

ou (puissance ocre granuleuse du continu)
sortir de lui-même en myriades émerveillantes d'intermédiaires

— là où nous (H. et moi) avons été appelés là un dimanche matin (en quel froid début de printemps ?), par G., correspondant du *Monde* à Orléans, non loin d'un établissement où de vieux Maghrébins sans famille
vivent leur retraite —

combien sont-ils à s'être réfugiés — clandestins —
et à s'entasser, la nuit, dans d'étroits édicules en béton (probablement des cabanes de jardins ouvriers abandonnés) ?
La plupart **nous regardent**, debout, **en silence**…

Il y a là — nous l'apprenons sans avoir demandé les identités ou appartenances — quelques Algériens, un Égyptien, des Africains (une femme, une seule, logée — nous montre-t-on, en ouvrant l'une des cabanes… matelas et couvertures entassés… — avec l'un des hommes). Et se font connaître (par l'intermédiaire de l'Égyptien) quelques jeunes hommes du Darfour.

On erre un peu (sacs ou bouteilles en plastique dans les herbes, inévitablement, papiers, matelas pourris)… sans réclamer, certes, de tout voir.

Pas de point d'eau, constatons-nous.
Il semble que celui qui, à quelques centaines de mètres de là, au bord de la route, aurait pu être utilisé, a été fermé — sur l'initiative de quelle autorité ? par quelle décision de les dissuader de rester là ?
Que boivent-ils ? Ce que des membres d'associations leur donnent, avec de la nourriture.

> Dans l'énorme bidonville de Nanterre, durant les années 60-61,
> au bord d'une route « nationale » (voitures, le dimanche soir),
> (champs de boue sans aucune installation, baraques édifiées de débris, bouts de planches, cartons, tôles et tissus)
> (et aussi : menaces [contradictoires], contrôles… couvre-feu, tirs, dans la nuit, à « balles réelles »)

> c'était, pour les enfants,
> un long chemin
> jusqu'à l'unique point d'eau accessible
> — au-delà, juste, de « leur » espace, de cet « entre »-là malgré tout, frustement,
> constitué là —

avec de petites carrioles
à grandes roues à traîner et pousser dans les ornières puantes,
et de lourds bidons en alu
(récupérés dans d'archaïques épiceries d'« arabes »)

Pour se laver (et leurs vêtements), ils ont l'eau de la Loire :
« on… » (un Algérien traduit pour tous — même s'il avoue mal comprendre l'arabe des gens du Darfour), « on sent mauvais »…
et ils nous font, en effet, sentir, non sans manifester par gestes leur humiliation, l'aigreur qu'exhalent les plis de leurs vêtements imprégnés des particules de boue
(celle qui — sur les plans d'eau glissant tournoyant ou dans les torsions et malgré les arrachements soudain blancs — brunit le fleuve.)

Au moment où nous remontons en voiture, deux des plus jeunes, assis sur une borne au bord de la route, nous suivent expressivement du regard.
Puisqu'ils semblent nous avoir attendus là, nous allons vers eux (et d'autres alors s'approchent, interviennent, traduisent encore un peu, maladroitement.)
L'un des deux se plaint de fièvre, de douleurs à la tête. L'autre retrousse une manche, montre son avant-bras : partout de petites élevures, j'y passe le bout du doigt. La gale ?

« Une recrudescence de maladies ! »
« la tuberculose, la gale »
(Propos de l'adjoint à la sécurité de la mairie d'Orléans)

C'est un dimanche après-midi, et à l'hôpital, où nous les emmenons, on refuse — poliment — de les examiner.
Chez un médecin de garde (dans un faubourg), la salle d'attente est pleine : femmes avec de petits enfants (otites).

On attend.
Avec l'un des deux,
qui parle un peu d'anglais (appris, dit-il, en écoutant la radio),
je vais dans le couloir ;

son père, éleveur, a (raconte-t-il en tâtonnant) été tué
et sa mère (après que des miliciens l'eurent sommé de se joindre à eux
sous peine d'être abattu)
l'a poussé à fuir
(restant, elle, seule avec ses sœurs).

Et puis… on entre à cinq (eux deux, G., H. et moi) dans le cabinet.
Le médecin, jeune, visiblement épuisé (cris de petits), proteste (« ce n'est pas un salon
ici »), manifeste (dès qu'il comprend que les deux consultants relèvent de la CMU) sa
mauvaise humeur (sans aller, comme
d'autres, jusqu'à refuser de les examiner) et après quelques phrases
qui auront suffi pour qu'il se radoucisse, il ausculte, palpe, rédige des ordonnances.

Et suivront, bien sûr (jours, semaines, voire mois)
nombre d'autres épisodes, pharmacie, laverie, argent, etc.
puis… d'autres interventions,
dont celle, finalement — inquiétante —,
de l'administration…

(« *Il y en a !* »
C'est un infirmier qui crie — dans le monde de la Kolyma, où survit
Chalamov parmi des centaines de milliers de zeks.
« 'Il y en a, Lidia Ivanovna !', dit-il,
et il cria à Andréiev : 'Pourquoi es-tu couvert de poux, hein ?'
Mais la doctoresse ne le laissa pas continuer.
'Est-ce de leur faute ?', dit-elle à voix basse et d'un ton plein de reproches,
en appuyant sur le mot 'leur', et elle prit son stéthoscope sur la table. »)

Quelques semaines plus tard, on apprendra
que deux de ces hommes (du Darfour), revenant de la ville vers « leur »
bord de Loire, et traversant dans la nuit les voies du pont de chemin de fer,
ont été écrasés.

> (L'entrefilet dans le journal local mentionnait que les « papiers » de l'un d'eux avaient
> pu être ramassés…, et qu'on aurait prévenu sa famille [?])

Le Monde du 11 octobre 2006 (du correspondant à Nairobi) :
« Au Darfour, la trêve du Ramadan a vécu. Alors que le gouvernement soudanais, depuis trois mois, a massé des troupes dans cette région, vaste comme la France, de l'ouest du pays et recruté de nouveaux miliciens, une offensive d'envergure contre les rebelles et la population du Darfour semble imminente. [...]
Un récit de l'extrême violence ordinaire au Darfour a été rendu public, lundi, par le Haut-Commissariat des Nations Unies pour les droits de l'homme, décrivant une série d'attaques contre le village de Buram, au sud du Darfour, entre le 28 août et le 1er septembre. L'attaque, menée par des miliciens recrutés au sein des tribus « arabes » par les forces de sécurité soudanaises, aurait fait des centaines de morts civils. Aucun rebelle n'était, semble-t-il, présent à Buram. Les Nations Unies mettent en avant la responsabilité du gouvernement soudanais dans ce massacre, tout en demandant qu'une enquête soit réalisée pour en identifier les auteurs. »

SE LAISSER ARRÊTER ou plutôt
ÊTRE (« nous ») INTERROMPU — par ce qui vient du bord, ou d'au-delà du bord…, par ce qui se trouve soudain passer au milieu du « dans » ?
Pouvoir être interrompu : générosité, liberté… ?

Cependant, **pour vivre des irruptions**

> *par coups de fil n'importe quand, alertes par email…*
> *ou simplement :* **en acceptant***, dans la rue, à la télé,* ***de voir***
> ***ce qu'on n'avait pas prévu de voir****,*
> *— et de manière, s'il se peut, à*
> ***en tirer des conséquences****…*

ne faut-il pas **être assez continu,**
disposer de suffisamment de forces pour
ne pas craindre d'y être exposé ?

    Car les interruptions du fait de la misère sont purement stériles : rien
que les enchevêtrements de vies dès lors confuses
<small>(cris, passages se jetant à travers, musiques s'entrecoupant, signaux de défis, publicités,
réclamations sans fin, insultes)</small>

rien qu'impossibilité (instable, nerveuse) de former des visées durables,
…rien d'autre qu'impuissance
<small>(voire, vite — multiplications de haines…)</small>

<small>Est-ce seulement à qui est</small> **ici de droit**
dans l'élément (fût-il équivoque) du « dans »,
<small>qu'il est permis de pouvoir
(droit ? bonheur ? angoisse ?)</small>
être interrompu par ce qui
<small>(ceux qui)</small>
se trouvera <small>(trouveront)</small>
faire irruption
<small>brisant (une infra-seconde) toute visée…
comme, à travers des feuillages,
gerbes, éclaboussures…</small>
sang psychique

Bleue, simplement, cendreuse, apparemment calme, vers 18 heures (novembre ?)
la place de la Poste
(un endroit presque central, mais un peu en décalage, dans la ville)
(de là part une rue où les Noirs, les Turcs, sont de plus en plus nombreux) (la mairie semble manœuvrer pour les repousser plus loin…)

refaite il y a peut-être trente ans, gros édifice terne
<small>comme en transparence,
pour quelqu'un né comme moi pendant la guerre,
palpite le souvenir d'une couleur, celle, acide-heureuse, du massif cube de briques
qu'était encore la Poste après la guerre, ayant survécu aux bombardements de 44
— non loin de décombres blancs, d'éventrements de la ville jusqu'aux caves
(eaux vertes, dans des plâtras sous le ciel, des années durant)</small>

Au milieu, une étendue de laid gazon, dalles synthétiques, une ligne de tram, quelques bancs. Douceur — avec quel goût métallique ?

> *De l'autre côté de la place, la Sécurité Sociale, quelques bancs,*
> *de vieux Maghrébins (à certaines heures)…*

La Poste (parvis de dalles synthétiques humides brillant grises vaguement orangées) n'est pas encore fermée (lumière par les portes vitrées).
Des Noirs, africains — probablement — (pas mal de femmes, des enfants poursuivant les pigeons) sont rassemblés, par petits groupes, dans le froid d'automne…

Je sors d'une petite agence de voyage tiède où j'ai pris un billet pour les États-Unis.

Papiers miens (passeport, cette fois-ci, avec visa de travail, lettre sur papier pelure, etc. : « documents » — objets de précautions légèrement fiévreuses — mêlant, dans les poches, leur odeur à celle des vêtements, de la sueur).
Papiers leurs. « Leurs » ? je n'ai aucune raison de supposer, à vrai dire, qu'ils sont les uns et les autres dans des situations équivalentes. Quoi qu'il en soit, la poste (les guichets), c'est pour tous le lieu des livrets, des mandats, c'est le support des liens avec là-bas…

> *Sur l'un des bords de la place, **un tram***
> *s'est arrêté dans l'obscurité peu à peu venue, il **repart***
> *(pour s'enfoncer dans plusieurs kilomètres de banlieue)*
> *éclairé du dedans,*
> *corps entassés, côte-à côte, face-à-face — veillant à s'ignorer.*
> *S'il court pourtant **de la quasi-attention***
> *(dont chaque visage, comme léché par un reflet de flamme,*
> *peut être fugitivement*
> *le support),*
> *c'est non pas des uns pour les autres mais **pour***
> ***ce qui,** entre tous, ne peut être tout à fait contenu,*
> *et **brûle**.*

« JE NE DEVRAIS PAS ÊTRE LÀ »
(là — hors de tout « dans » … ?)

C'est à tort, bien sûr
(en agglomérant, par une bêtise très partagée, facilitante, trop d'« autres » en masses,
là où
pourtant les distinctions sont vitales),
que, rêvassant (à l'abri), **j'aurai**, *un instant,*
lisant un peu plus tard (chez moi, donc) Judith Soussan
(son livre découvert par internet m'accompagne au moins par intermittences),
attribué cette voix
à l'un quelconque *de ceux que j'essayais de me faire revoir*
(mais devenus déjà trop mêlés dans ma mémoire)
tels qu'ils étaient — **sur la place de la Poste.**

« Je ne devrais pas être là »… Ce propos est tenu par Désiré, un SDF africain. Il a été recueilli, donc, dans *Les SDF africains en France*.

Judith Soussan a écouté, transcrit, et, dans ses réflexions, elle accueille, à sa façon, ces paroles de gens qui sont « à la marge ».
« Cette 'marge' », remarque-t-elle calmement, « peut nous éclairer. »

« …Parce que dans ma tête c'est ouvert et je sais pas quoi prendre … »
Ces mots-là, transcrits ailleurs dans le livre, sont ceux d'un autre SDF africain : Cyprien.

Prendre quelque chose — ce à quoi se tenir en dépit de tout, une idée pour orienter sa vie — dans sa tête ?

Si **« c'est ouvert »**, Cyprien a-t-il encore un **« dans »** sa tête ?
Sa tête (se dira le lecteur des propos de Cyprien), peut-être est-elle ouverte parce qu'il n'a **rien dans quoi être,** parce que **rien ne l'enveloppe.**

Pour être en mesure de saisir ses propres pensées — ou ne serait-ce que
ses sensations et émotions, ses désirs, ou un minimum d'espoir —
faut-il être **dans** quelque chose ?

Est-il donc nécessaire
d'appartenir,
ne peut-on se rapporter à soi
qu'en se sachant contenu
dans ?

Un seul « dans » ?
ou des « dans » concentriques, se renforçant
(orbes de chaleur rougissant, pour quel flair, l'air des rues) ?

ou complexes, intersectés, se révélant incohérents ?
voire incompatibles, à la folie,
jusqu'à vibrer s'entrebriser
(enveloppes comme de verre, dans le vide,
arêtes absurdes, sanglantes)

Être — se reconnaître — s'identifier … comme quoi ? SDF ? sans papiers ?
Cyprien (écouté par Judith Soussan) : « Je me sentais même pas là-dedans ».

Judith Soussan prête attention à ce qui se différencie, voire s'oppose, dans ces marges mal vues par la plupart d'entre « nous ».
Et aussi, elle donne accès à ce que chacun essaie de penser de sa position…

Nuances dans les catégorisations (sociologiques ? administratives ? juridiques ?)…
Ou plutôt, entre SDF et sans papiers : différence entre des caractérisations respectivement économique et politique ? ou (également) entre ce dont on pourrait être tenu pour responsable et ce dont on ne peut s'imputer la faute à soi-même ?

Cyprien : « Ça m'a fait rien du tout, parce que c'est ce que j'ai pas voulu, il y avait une seule chose qui me bloquait, c'était les papiers, et pour moi c'était pas ma faute. »
Et il insiste : « Il y avait aucun sentiment de culpabilité… je me sentais pas concerné. »

(Pourquoi a-t-il remarqué, au passage : « Avant le mot 'sans-papiers', il y avait 'étrangers en situation irrégulière'… » ?)

Cyprien : qu'est-ce qu'avoir la tête ouverte et qu'en sentir le « contenu » se perdre dans le vide — en pointillements qui, ni dedans ni dehors, grésillent, se dispersent ?

Dans quel endroit (la rue, une place peut-être *comme celle de la Poste*, le bord d'un fleuve, un squat),
ne pouvoir alimenter, de toutes ses forces,
qu'**une hémorragie de points** aveuglants :
rien que micro-palpitations de l'incompréhensible, dans le temps qui se perd ?

Dans quoi penser, le soir, au moment d'aller dormir — **ou le matin**, en allant où… ?

Mais Cyprien ou Désiré (nourris, vêtus, abrités)…, au moins « appartiennent »-ils à ce « dans » minimum que voudrait constituer Emmaüs.

Communiqué de Presse (Paris, le 22 mars 2006)
« […] Le mouvement Emmaüs France, réunissant plus de 250 structures d'accueil et d'accompagnement de personnes en difficultés, exprime sa vive inquiétude concernant l'avant-projet de loi du 9 février modifiant le code de l'entrée et du séjour des étrangers et du droit d'asile (CESEDA), et la circulaire du 21 février intitulée « Conditions de l'interpellation d'un étranger en situation irrégulière, garde à vue de l'étranger en situation irrégulière, réponses pénales » diffusée aux préfets par le Ministère de l'intérieur.
Les groupes Emmaüs accueillent en moyenne 20 à 25% d'étrangers en leur sein. Elles considèrent le fait d'accueillir toutes les personnes avec les mêmes droits et devoirs et sans critère de sélection à l'entrée, comme deux conditions fondamentales de leur intégration et du développement de leurs talents. »

LE « DANS » même : À SENTIR (saveur sauvage) — où ? quand ? par ou pour qui ? —

Le ressentir aux instants, bruts, où il se révèle condition déchirée,
menaçante,
du sentir…

> *… avec, toujours, l'imminence*
> *de sa destruction possible*
> (comme jadis, en temps de guerre, maisons à vitres bleues,
> vibrations sous un ciel envahi
> d'objets monstrueux)

Se sentir APPARTENIR, et comme infusé du « DANS » ?

éclat spécial (par exemple dans les aéroports)
— soudain dangereux ? —
de ceux qui, y compris hors de « chez eux » (commerce, tourisme),
relèvent d'un état protecteur,
qui, sans y songer,
se sentent tels à tout instant

Est-ce obéir-croire à du politiquement décidé — du circonscrivant (contenant) et excluant ?

> Une société politique serait-elle à vivre
> comme un « système social complet et fermé » ?
> « Complet, parce qu'il se suffit à soi-même,
> et offre de la place à toutes les finalités importantes de la vie.
> Fermé, parce que les seules façons d'y entrer et d'en sortir
> sont la naissance ou la mort. » (Rawls)
>
> Mais Lefort :
> **« …on ne saurait localiser l'homme 'dans' la société… »**

Im-migrer : passer — se sentir passer (se deviner vu passer) — **dans** quoi ?

        Dans quelle visibilité commune — ici, à Orléans, par exemple —
        se savoir su ? avec hostilité ? ou essayer d'y rester ignoré ?

Dans quel élément implicite et puissant (disponibilité poudroyante de l'entre) espérer être pris en compte ? Réussir, compter, marquer — ou, en avançant, possibiliser l'air même ?

Mais, tout en risquant ici (espérant, redoutant) une visibilité nouvelle (pour l'administration, ou dans les regards-idées des gens),
s'acharner, coûteusement (jusqu'à l'épuisement), à ne pas cesser de
compter — d'être quasi visible, imaginé, espéré —
pour ceux qui sont restés **là-bas** (et qui attendent, ont besoin, comptent sur…).

Devoir (audacieux ? accablé ?) vivre (non, parfois, sans forfanterie et faux-semblants, ou, hélas, jusqu'à l'amertume… années, fatigue, chute) dans **deux** « **dans** » (…reliés par mandats, coups de téléphone) ?

Que savons-nous (sentons-pensons), « nous » (assurés de nos places au sein d'un — plusieurs ? — « dans »),
de « leurs » raisons de partir ?

« La spirale du rejet [*qui parle là ? j'ai perdu… recopié sur internet puis perdu… ça vient de* Cultures et conflits] s'amorce avec une histoire : le demandeur d'asile raconte ce qui l'a conduit à quitter son pays et cette relation écrite ou orale est difficile et, nécessairement, longue… »
« Même l'explication d'un départ hâtif parcourt plusieurs années de vie : soit parce que la situation de l'exilé s'est détériorée insidieusement jusqu'à un stade, subjectivement perçu, de crainte rédhibitoire ; soit parce que le facteur déclencheur aussi prompt soit-il n'économise pas ultérieurement à l'exilé la peine de remonter loin dans le temps pour s'expliquer à lui-même d'abord, et aux autres ensuite, cet étrange basculement dans sa vie ; soit enfin parce que la société chaotique qui pousse à l'exil recèle une complexité difficile à maîtriser […] »

« … les formulaires des procédures d'asile ne font pas place à une telle expansion […]. Les rejets sont massifs, la procédure expéditive et inquisitoriale. Le demandeur s'expose d'abord par écrit et en quelques pages. Le récit est bref, sec, improvisé sur un coin de guichet, sous la pression d'une file d'attente, handicapé par le recours à un intermédiaire […] »
« Viennent ensuite les phases d'audition », « le même constat de collision entre les temps d'écoute et la possibilité pour l'exilé de se faire comprendre. »

Qui, de nous (et, prétendument, « pour nous »), écoute ces paroles ? Contrôle administratif (d'où papiers, dossiers, comptes-rendus, surveillance, arrestations, expulsions)

Qui, de nous (pour nous ?) cherche à percevoir et analyser cette écoute ? « Scientifiquement » ? Politiquement ?
(d'où articles, livres, émissions, interventions — parfois —)

Qui surveille ? Qui surveille la surveillance ?
Des personnes presque identiques, de formations sûrement voisines —
mais entre lesquelles il arrive que tout « nous » doive se déchirer.

QUI, DE NOUS, QUOI, EN NOUS, à travers les uns ou les autres,
QUEL NOUS-ATTENTION, QUEL REGARD-INSTANCE,

était présupposé, espéré,
cherché

quel « nous »
valant comme autre puissant
qu'espéreraient (réclameraient — jusqu'à, parfois, le haïr)
des centaines de milliers d'abandonnés ?

par ce reportage télé

> *— qui, en même temps qu'il sait*
> *trouver ce qu'il nous fait voir, fouille vers nous (qu'il anticipe)…*
> *à l'initiative de qui (et avec quelles informations préalables)*
> *le projet fut-il formé, et avec quels moyens, donnés par qui, fut-il réalisé ?*

sur des enfants-esclaves au Ghana, achetés par des pêcheurs, à cinq ou six ans, à peine nourris, en guenilles, battus… ?

L'un (ayant constaté que d'autres ont été rachetés par une association et que lui n'a pu l'être) est vu pleurant,
de profil, visage contre le lac,

vu plus que seul, mais, là, cette fois, à coup sûr, **se sachant vu,**
s'étant, donc, senti, mais pour combien de minutes,
su

puis — quoi ?

> Et pour les « rachetés », qu'apercevons-nous de leurs parents
> — par qui ils ont (moins petits poucets abandonnés que corps
> négociables)
> bien des chances d'être revendus ?
> *(Un faux — prématuré — vieillard, riant édenté,*
> *au milieu de ce qui ne parvient pas à être un village,*
> *se vante*
> *d'avoir fait vingt enfants et d'en avoir vendu cinq.)*

> Et, de ceux qui les achètent,
> que voyons-nous ?

Un long maigre bras de femme sort de derrière une toile
(sur un marché),
agrippe un enfant, l'éloigne de « nos » regards :
« cet enfant est à moi ! »,
« elle ment », chuchote le guide-traducteur (un homme du pays,
vaguement moqueur),
« c'est un enfant-esclave ».

Et d'où, quand, pour « nous » (de loin ou déjà dans la ville), **va-t-elle encore
fuser,** inattendue, obsédante,
la question

celle **du bord**
faisant irruption, éclair à goût d'encre,
au milieu...
disjoignant toute réalisation de **notre prétendu « dans »,**

le trouvant soudain là où, brûlant, il ne
tient pas en lui-même...,

sous quel angle se redécochera-t-elle,
**de quels coins ou replis
du dehors-dedans,**

de quels nœuds de difficultés et solutions à entretenir
(ainsi de là où, en plein midi,
sur la place du Martroi, entre banques, chambre de commerce, cafés,
dans une manifestation pour les
sans-papiers où se trouvaient rassemblés des membres — une petite centaine —

              d'associations, des parents d'élèves, etc.,
               H., allant de l'un ou l'une à l'autre,
a trouvé une promesse d'embauche pour M. O., congolais en quête de papiers)
                ou relancée à partir de
        quels mauvais dérobements de l'entrevisibilité
         (ces lieux ou minutes où certains, en pleine lumière,
           sont imperceptibles ou, au contraire,
            échouent cruellement à ne pas être vus :
cet homme, par exemple, remis — à une station de tram éclairée (22 heures) près de
laquelle nous passons — entre les mains de policiers (qui le menottent)
par un contrôleur qui a constaté qu'il était dépourvu non seulement de
« titre de transport » mais de papiers…
… une femme (cinquante ans ?) ivre ou folle, ou simplement à bout…,
descendue du tram et punie d'une amende,
crie depuis le bord du trottoir, supplie qu'on lâche l'homme (qu'elle ne connaît pas),
hulule sanglots et imprécations…
Et nous (H. et moi) ? Nous nous inquiétons, nous insérons, demandons, harcelons… :
« si voulez savoir ce qui se passe », dit l'un des flics, « engagez-vous dans la police… »

**DIRE-EFFECTUER UN INSTANT — LE « NOUS », LE « DANS » MÊME : seules
le pourraient des phrases dont la nécessité** (l'impulsion formatrice) **renaîtrait toujours
par éruption interne ou du dehors, de ce qui laboure ce « dans » d'obscurité,** le sillonne
d'une fluidité d'une trop crue fraîcheur,

phrases déroulées noires-poreuses résorbant à mesure l'attention,

formulations auto-dévoratrices imposées par les instants-endroits où, en plein « dans »,
se recrée

du non enveloppable, du fait de divisions toujours recréées, celles du trop loin-trop proche,
celles de doublures enflammées d'incompatibilité, ou **de l'inappropriable,** nécessairement
disputé par plusieurs, dans un jeu trop sérieux, arrachements vite sanglants,

mais aussi, indissociablement, **du disputé de soi à soi,** du temps-substance-soi déroulé en
changements d'états (de l'« ordinaire » à quelles excitations, rages, évanouissements sexuels,
lieux-moments féroces des corps), ou accidenté en absorptions (passions, dépendances
absolues), dénivellations (sursauts incontrôlables du sentir, décalages et chutes noirâtres
des pensées)

et encore, subreptices, tout le temps, lumineux, vitalement odorants et perlants de sucs,
des contacts, **alliages chairs-choses,** alliances ou soutiens (humains, plantes, animaux, etc.
— tout cela toujours au bord de se broyer, catastrophique…)

Vivant (visible ? invisible ?) dans le bord, dans l'épaisseur même du bord
Laura (une trentaine d'années, deux enfants) ?

> (**Pourquoi a-t-elle fui l'Angola ?** Elle a cru l'expliquer devant
> diverses instances…
> À l'une, quasi ultime, H. a assisté ; les membres de cette commission de recours ont paru
> ébranlés…, émus !
> H. s'était dite, au retour, presque sûre d'une réponse enfin positive…
> Et puis — refus. Pour s'en tenir à des chiffres fixés par le ministère ?)

Laura, donc,
il y a quelques mois, séparée pour quelque temps de ses enfants
(par prudence),
avait été hébergée (« protégée ») ici, « à la maison »

> (avant que, défendue, et comme revendiquée, contre la préfecture par un maire UDF
> de banlieue, elle ne soit logée dans un bâtiment de l'hôpital psychiatrique au bord de
> la forêt et qu'elle obtienne enfin des papiers — temporaires, il est vrai),

et j'essayais, en parlant, de lui faire oublier son angoisse

> (mains s'agitant, lèvres blanchies :
> par terreur de « la DDASS » qui, pleurait-elle,
> allait lui « prendre » son garçon de six ans et sa fille de quatre ans)

ainsi m'a-t-elle raconté comment il lui était arrivé
(du fait qu'il lui fallait quitter dès le matin l'hébergement d'urgence où elle avait trouvé refuge)
de passer, avec sa fille (le garçon étant à l'école),
des heures, en hiver, **dans la tiédeur éclairée des abords d'une** démesurée **« grande surface »**

> (la seule. semble-t-il, qui ait pu — grâce à quelles « influences » ? — s'installer
> au centre d'Orléans),

sans accéder, donc, au magasin même (comment payer quoi que ce soit ?),
mais en se cantonnant à la marge des caisses (là où évoluent, très
visibles, en chemise blanche, des vigiles — noirs pour la plupart…),
usant les heures, avec sa fillette,
abritées, l'une et l'autre, fût-ce juste au bord, par cette carcasse de baleine métallique…

et elle n'était pas la seule, m'a-t-elle expliqué…
d'autres erraient là, silencieux (sauf incidents)

elle, comme tous ces marginaux, étant **visible**, évidemment, mais **sans être**
(par tolérance ? ne comptant pas pour les caméras ?) **vue,**
juste **au bord**
de ce très pauvre **palais de la visibilité**
(celle que se disputent les produits :
emballages — cartons, plastiques, cellophanes —, couleurs calculées, contacts,
odeurs de « propre », ou du douceâtre, ou de l' acide, ou l'huile comme plissée dans les
cannelures des bouteilles
produits brillant d'émulation pour paraître exactement ceux « faits pour »
(« pour », un instant, telle bande de gamines souples luisantes ricanières avides, tout
autant que de choses, de leur propre entrevisibilité dans les files aux caisses),
ceux devenant toujours plus ce qui serait de toujours attendu
comme du sucre qui fondrait, exact, sans reste,
dans la nuit du goût

Et lui encore, DANS SA TÊTE,
qu'est-ce qu'il pouvait bien avoir,
que pouvait-il bien « se dire »,

ce type, rue de la République ?

mais moi, aussi bien,
est-ce qu'à cet instant (courant à demi) je formais des phrases **dans ma tête** ?

…des mi-mots, peut-être, oui, de la mousse
d'enthousiasme sous l'effet du soleil horizontal sur la Loire
héron ardoisé replié de froid,
aigrette — éblouissante-éblouie dans la lumière ? —
sortant, à pas précautionneux mais soudain accélérés,
d'entre des touffes jaunies prises dans la glace…
(« pour » personne,
ces vies surprises avec excitation
comme un secret sexuel de la « nature » ?)

Il était là, ce matin de novembre (en plein sur mon chemin vers la gare), homme noir (d'âge incertain),
debout au milieu de la rue

>(la plus commerçante, la seule du centre à être hantée par des jeunes venus des banlieues)

homme gelé

sorti d'où dans la préaube ?

> *bizarrement,*
> *il ne lui avait donc pas (pas encore ? il faisait à peine jour...)*
> *été interdit d'être là*
> *— malgré tous les arrêtés pris à Orléans*
> *pour que nul ne rencontre que du*
> *prévu*

> tombé d'où, donc, et comment ?
> c'était peu après des émeutes, des caillassages :
> trams et bus de nuit supprimés, chaos, peut-être voulu, des communications
> avec la banlieue

> **L'été précédent,**
> je l'avais aperçu à plusieurs reprises, dans cette même rue,
> errant en pleine foule, longuement arrêté, ou assis, parfois, sur un banc
> à un arrêt de tram, chargé de paquets mal ficelés dépenaillés,
> excoriés-cotonneux,
> en plein soleil, au milieu de jeunes (nonchalants, ou traversés de
> vagues d'excitation)

> une fois il m'avait paru (non loin de la FNAC, devant un magasin de vêtements)
> être entré, confusément, en conversation
> avec quelques-uns,
> des Noirs ? des Beurs ? ou, aussi, de ces blonds translucides du nord (descendants
> d'immigrés polonais ?),

> la plupart habillés d'une manière, bien entendu, codée mais non
> sans qu'elle puisse se faire inattendue, jaillissante...
> ils ne se moquaient pas — pas vraiment...
> plutôt incrédules, interrompus dans leur avidité de voir être vus,
> ils semblaient plutôt stupéfaits, ou inquiets
> — sur ce bord de la visibilité

moins de trente ans, sans doute — longues mèches laineuses noires brunâtres (tressées d'elles-mêmes par l'absence de soins, ou bien restes d'une coiffure élaborée...)

> le ***décrire*** ?
> *lui donner, ici, l'attention qu'il détruisait ?*

à présent debout dans le jour qui se levait à peine, dans le vent glacial d'un carrefour,

immobile raidi (incapable désormais de s'asseoir) au milieu des gens pressés (chacun courant dans sa propre visibilité anticipée, celle d'une journée à vivre)

obtuse étrave fichée au milieu du flux

ses paquets (les mêmes depuis l'été passé ?) empilés près de lui
> dans les jambes, quasiment,
> de ceux qui les découvraient soudain sur le sol de dalles grises

un pain trempé, ficelé au flanc d'un des ballots, et faisant saillie dans le passage

et **lui pyramidal**
comme fait des plis du plastique transparent déchiré dont il avait essayé de s'envelopper,
ou des écorces-épaisseurs, débordantes, de ses vêtements superposés hétéroclites
certains vestiges entrevus magnifiques, bouts de quelles défroques...,
du cuir, des pans d'étoffes éclatantes, morceaux d'où prélevés, pour
de théâtrales chamarrures, pour une présentation hallucinatoire d'un soi pourrissant

tant **d'amas** humides contre le froid, ou contre... quoi ?
apotropaïques comme des cris ? des torsions de main ? dans le vide

et dessous quel corps mal imaginable ? en quel état ?
et **dans**
sa tête ? quoi ?
quels mots en attente ? ou ... mi-mots

                est-ce qu'il se faisait, encore, des promesses de « m'en sortir », est-ce qu'il
                            pouvait encore se dire qu'il n'était *pas*
                                      ce qu'il était
                                                là ...

                  (et si ç'avait été un matin un de mes enfants, découvert là, et tel, à
                                l'issue d'une nuit pareille — que ...)

il ne tendait pas la main
n'avait pas à côté de lui, comme d'autres (cette femme mendiante — asiatique, exceptionnellement — toujours sur le même seuil, un peu plus loin, mais à d'autres heures), **un gobelet en plastique** où il aurait mis quelques pièces pour amorcer les dons

et ... à l'instant où je

                                                      raconter ça ?
                              avoir cru pouvoir rapporter ça, enfantinement, à la maison ...

bute sur ses paquets, il tousse, visage dont de l'eau s'exprime, crache

ai-je été éclaboussé — et ... inquiet ... — d'être souillé ? contaminé ?

à peine l'ai-je dépassé je ne peux — *par quoi accroché et durement ramené ?* — que rebrousser
et (cherchant une pièce dans ma poche)
m'adresser à lui : « vous ... vous avez besoin ... ? » « de ... ? »

ses paupières quasi-closes collées de secrétions s'entr'ouvrent péniblement laissant voir le blanc (sous les iris) de globes à demi chavirés de ses lèvres un ahanement faible — un rire ? —

il ruisselle il fume *condensant-décomposant l'air entre nos visages*
il exhale le dégel du brouillard qui, toute la nuit, avait gelé sur lui

auréole d'ammoniac
de l'urine qui a transpercé ses enveloppes,
bave sur la barbe floconneuse

je touche sa main brusquement (sans qu'il dise un mot) apparue

que serait-ce (peur d'une seconde)
*si **cette main alors** m'agrippait*
(au moment où je vais prendre « mon train »)
et si soudain là
se concrétisait impérieusement le lien
que de toujours on a su pouvoir — devoir ? — se créer avec celui à qui on a donné,
une redoutable (dévoratrice ?) dépendance

mais
maintenant, ici, hé bien — je me...
suis un peu perdu, je lâche prise

je ne sais plus ce qu'ici, il aurait fallu formuler, quelles précisions...
ni pourquoi

cet homme — plus que seul, « désaffilié » — était-il forcément un **sans-papiers ?**

SDF, oui, clandestin, peut-être pas

les distinctions entre situations peuvent être décisives
et d'abord (Judith Soussan) vitales « dans » une « tête »
celle, là, de cet homme gelé,
durant, surtout, ces heures où peut-être il essayait de... « se parler »
— en pleine rue ce matin-là —

absorbé à maintenir sa continuité
— « dans » ? « hors » ?

et donc si..., dans ces phrases, je tendais à
un argument politique, est-ce que je viens de le perdre
et n'aurais-je fait que le renoyer dans
ce qui s'est réimposé, submergeant, des sensations mi-pensées
de la rue ?

Je l'ai revu une fois en décembre devant la Poste
(à distance des groupes d'Africains)

adossé, un soir, au mur, un seul ballot, rouleau blanchâtre (couchage ?),
coincé derrière lui,
il jouait du pipeau (trouvé où ?)
en tapant, sur les dalles du parvis encore éclairées par un reste de jour,
d'un pied
sans paraître voir personne
sans regard

tenant une pièce dans la main je lui ai donné, du haut du bras,
une légère poussée
de côté
et de nouveau sa main s'est, à peine, tendue
et j'ai effleuré ses doigts de
cuir brun-orangé crevassé

puis plus jamais

OU ENCORE, *mais vite, il est trop tard (le temps est épuisé)*

COMME UN COUP À (ou un **agrippement sur**) **L'ÉPAULE,**
me forçant à me retourner sur ce qui était en train d'avoir lieu, dans mon dos, à Roissy (alors que je venais de passer — guérites en verre — le contrôle des papiers
pressé, comme chacun, de me disjoindre de la masse des passagers du même avion,

qu'est-ce qui m'a pris ?

Ce fut (retour de Pékin, quelques collègues sortis avant moi me faisant de loin déjà des signes d'adieu)
non pas exactement, à coup sûr, **une affaire de sans-papiers,**
mais plutôt celle de papiers insuffisants... [?],

de quoi bloquer là
celui qui, pendant le voyage, avait été mon voisin

                                        onze heures durant
              j'avais été assis — au milieu, exclusivement, de Chinois
                    qui semblaient plus ou moins organisés en groupe
                         (naïf, peut-être, qu'est-ce que je ne voyais pas ?) —
                                                              à côté de lui

                         voisin de gauche (près du hublot)
                         (raide veste brune, mains rondes, visage épais grêlé),
                         au moment du repas (sur Air France),
                         son pain, qu'il ne sait comment se mettre dans la bouche,
                         je lui montre comment le rompre, etc.
                                              (*fraternisation !*)

mais je ne peux pas maintenant... dire, relâcher cette prise (elle ne cessera plus de me tenir)

simplement, **ce fut alors**
— soucieux (corps mien révulsé) de lui (arrêté là alors que je passais), imaginant son retour forcé, l'argent (de qui... ? perdu), le gâchis et (famille, village) l'humiliation —

ce fut...,
retournant vers le flic, contre lui,
passage, presque, « à l'acte » (vain ? ou pire ?)
crier réellement — et pourtant comme en rêve (s'éveillant au milieu de tous en train de réaliser son cauchemar) !

Y « reviendrai »-je ? **Rien**, ici, évidemment — ni les évidences perçantes, ni la confusion, ou l'aveuglement, **ni**
la question :
rien ne s'est apaisé, rien **ne s'arrête — là**

Notes

Du Darfour à la Loire avec Ousmane pour commencer

> Qui sollicite ton avis au sujet de cet étranger?
> Et si sans qu'on te le demande tu le donnes,
> alors va-t'en de nuit en nuit
> avec ses ulcères aux pieds, va! et ne reviens pas
> Ingeborg Bachmann

« **allez** » : il fait un geste du tranchant de la main dans l'air blanc.
Régulièrement, depuis des mois, nous parlons — dans la cuisine, en général. Lui ai-je fait croire que, sur les trois ou quatre récentes années de dénuement qu'il a vécues, nous pourrions, dès lors qu'il vit chez nous et que nous prenons le temps qu'il faut, rabattre jour après jour, des paroles, comme un pli apaisant de couverture ?

« **Allez vas-y.** » De sa voix, terreuse-amère, et du bras (silhouette sombre à contre-jour), il mime qui vous libère ou vous chasse. Dans une rue, naguère, en Libye. Ou, après une nuit de garde à vue, dans une rue de Paris ou d'Orléans. Ou à la porte d'un centre de rétention, au bord d'une route dans la forêt d'Orléans, à des kilomètres de tout (« Comment je fais ? » a-t-il dit au gendarme… « Pas mon problème… Allez vas-y. »)

« **Allez va…** » Il expulse dans l'air des phrases qui, depuis des mois, sont restées incluses en lui comme des dards.

Mais soudain c'est lui-même qui, debout devant la porte vitrée lumineuse, face à moi, s'adresse à lui-même ces mots : « **Allez vas-y.** »

« **Allez…** » Il n'a nulle part où aller, sinon cette famille « de blancs » (comme il m'a dit), cette maison où il habite depuis bientôt un an, cette cuisine…
Lui avons-nous donné de faux espoirs ? Papiers, travail : son ou notre impuissance — administrativement entretenue — a trop de chances d'être définitive.

« **Ici** », dit-il en se rasseyant lourdement, « **c'est pas la vie** » — ou (je transcris) « **pas-ma-la-vie.** »

« **Claude** », dit-il en regardant le carrelage gris, « **je vais partir.** » Vers où ? Pour risquer de disparaître dans une prison à Khartoum ? Ou, s'il en sort au bout de plusieurs mois, afin de tenter de retrouver sa mère, ses sœurs disparues… ou ne serait-ce que l'endroit dévasté de son village, ou les débris de sa maison ?

« **Ici** », martèle-t-il — et je n'aurai rien à lui répondre —, « **c'est pas-ma-la-vie.** »

*

Paroles d'Ousmane — ou « O. » —, exilé du Darfour…
Pourquoi avoir commencé par celles-ci — parmi tant d'autres que, de sa bouche, j'aurai entendues depuis près d'un an, et que je continue (au moment où j'achève ces lignes) d'entendre ?

Il les avait dites voilà des semaines… Mais elles étaient jusqu'alors restées en l'air — imminentes. Ce n'est que tout récemment — **20 mai 2008** — que je me suis résolu à les écrire — ou à les laisser, par mes mains, s'abattre, noires.

*

Noter ce que dit O., depuis bientôt un an qu'il habite ici et qu'il vient régulièrement parler — dans la cuisine, en fin d'après-midi —, j'ai scrupule à le faire pendant qu'il parle. Il hésite, il se heurte moins à des manques de vocabulaire ou aux défaillances de sa syntaxe qu'à sa rugueuse prononciation. Et puis soudain, ses phrases se bousculent, et voici que, sur la table encombrée (journaux, légumes, miettes), je ne trouve pas de papier ; j'attrape un bout de journal, ou une enveloppe déchirée, un crayon qui traîne — pour ne griffonner que mal, de côté, à la dérobée, gêné.

Et puis je répugne à l'interrompre. Ne faudrait-il pas, pourtant, reprononcer ses mots, ou lui retourner, recomposées, ses phrases ?

*

O. s'interrompt souvent lui-même, visage tourné vers le sol.
S'il relève soudain les yeux, je suis gêné d'être surpris à le regarder trop attentivement. Et que penserait-il s'il avait accès à des phrases qui, comme celles-ci, le décrivent ?

Il gratte de l'index le cadre en bois — grossier vernis qui pèle, fibres de pin — de la table (le plateau est de métal émaillé : mode d'il y a bien trente ans).

Bruits, alors, arrivant à travers les vitres — variant selon l'heure du jour ou la saison. Vent, clochette au coin du toit bas de la cuisine… Ou, par la porte entr'ouverte sur le jardin, cris d'aiguilles de mésanges… Ou…

Mais qu'est-ce qui, émanant de son existence si longtemps quasi muette comme de la mienne souvent verbeuse, s'épaissit au-dessus de la table, entre nos visages ? De l'impuissance double, redoublée.

*

Parfois, je lâche le crayon, renonce…
Je n'arrive plus à noter quand il arrive qu'à la tombée du jour (il va sortir : jamais il n'accepte de manger ici, il ira plutôt à une distribution de nourriture dans la rue, ou à un foyer, ou se fera lui-même une « petite cuisine »), il se mette à parler avec emportement.

Demain, au plus noir de la préaube, certaines de ses paroles, au-delà des ruptures du sommeil, réapparaîtront-elles, m'imposant de les transformer en phrases miennes… encore, il est vrai, à l'état d'ébauches ?

*

« Allez vas-y »… «…pas la vie », « pas-ma-la-vie… » : paroles épuisées d'impuissance, coups de la main ou du bras ou de la voix, contre quelles masses environnant de toute part…

Ces paroles-là,
pourquoi a-t-il fallu — au moment où (début mai 2008) j'ai entrepris de commencer à « fixer » (aigre et bête, ce mot) les notes que j'ai prises de nos conversations depuis bientôt un an — qu'elles me reviennent en pleine figure
 et

            au risque de me rendre incapable
        de remplir la promesse que je lui avais faite il y a des mois,
      celle de rendre un jour lisible — mais pour qui ? — ce qu'il dirait

> … sans, il est vrai, qu'il ait jamais l'air de se soucier
> de ce projet
> sinon, une fois, par une remarque peut-être ironique
> sur mes délais indéfinis — comparables (me suis-je dit vaguement amer)
> à ses rendez-vous parfois manqués, ses oublis ou
> négligences ?

m'arrêtent ?

*

20 mai 2008, donc : O. venait de rentrer avec un papier de la Préfecture (où — à tort, avions-nous jugé — il s'était rendu sans être accompagné) : un permis de séjour (« laissez-passer » dit-il) d'**un mois**.
Or, antérieurement, il recevait des permis de trois mois.

Pourquoi, ai-je pensé, cette réduction ? Qu'est-ce qui pouvait motiver cette soudaine restriction fabriquée par l'administration ?
J'ai alors imaginé (dans un accès, comme trop souvent, d'affolement inefficace, voire dangereux), que le processus engagé depuis quelques mois (après plus de deux années sans le moindre titre de séjour) allait s'interrompre… et quoi alors… expulsion… ?

Mais non, **trois jours après, O. a reçu une convocation pour la signature d'un « contrat d'intégration ».**

Restait pourtant que, dans ce papier (que je lui lisais faute qu'il puisse le déchiffrer), on lui réclamait une fois de plus — mais peut-être n'était-ce qu'automaticité des formulaires ou rituels administratifs — un passeport.

Chez lui, m'a-t-il expliqué un jour (comme il a tenté de faire pour l'administration), il n'a jamais eu de papiers. C'est à la ville qu'on avait des papiers. Dans son village (à cent cinquante kilomètres de Nyala), rien de pareil. Les identités n'avaient pas besoin d'être écrites. Un « vieux » se souvenait des gens, de chacun et de sa famille… Et si ce vieux-là venait à décliner ou quand il mourait, il y avait déjà un autre pour prendre le relais.

Aujourd'hui, cependant, a-t-il ajouté (sur le même ton âcre qui lui vient quand il constate l'impossibilité de rien savoir de ce qui, après sa fuite, est arrivé à sa famille — sa mère, ses sœurs, seules, sans homme), le vieux qui aurait pu se souvenir de lui n'avait-il pas disparu, déplacé ou mort — avec, peut-être, tout le village ?

*

Mais d'abord … pour commencer …
(tourbillons d'accès — il faudrait simultanément tout réouvrir)

qu'est-ce qui « prouve » qu'il est bien du Darfour ?

L'OFPRA, puis la commission de recours — en 2005 — n'ont pas ajouté foi à ses explications et assertions, lors d'auditions où l'interprète semble n'avoir pas bien compris son arabe, ou du moins sa prononciation…
Les attendus, sommaires, du refus incriminent sa manière de s'exprimer, jugée « stéréotypée ». A-t-on voulu insinuer que les précisions sur le Darfour par lesquelles il avait essayé de répondre à des questions soupçonneuses, auraient pu être recueillies par lui hors du Darfour — au Tchad, par exemple, parmi des réfugiés (foules, abords de quelque camp…) ?
(Ou bien — avatar grotesque de « notre » tradition oratoire et de « nos valeurs » — pour « réussir » devant ces commissions, les candidats à la régularisation auraient-ils à déployer un art de persuader qui, de surcroît, avec élégance, saurait se dissimuler comme tel ?)

*

« **T'as vu** » : **c'est souvent** (peu après être arrivé dans la cuisine) **par ces mots qu'il commence**, en s'asseyant face à moi (sous la lampe… la musique continue dans la pièce à côté), à raconter, à essayer d'expliquer…

« T'as vu … C'est pas-la-vie » …
Moins de vie (de droits, de possibles) que tous les autres ?

Avec tous les autres du Darfour qui comme lui s'étaient réfugiés au bord de la Loire, il avait été emmené dans un centre pour y attendre le résultat de l'examen de son dossier. Mais il est seul à ne pas avoir été régularisé. Vu autre, désormais, même par eux. Tombant hors.

*

NOTES

« *t'as vu…* » — être retombé, sans plus d'attache

dans les rues, tant de voix,
et des visages soudain sentis trop expressifs,

ou seul au bord du fleuve (toujours susceptible, pour qui survit dans les îles, de se
gonfler brun menaçant)

quand il pleut, la voûte en béton d'une arche du pont de chemin de fer,

et toujours chercher à manger dans les rues
et revenir s'endormir par terre

se laver, au réveil, dans l'eau terreuse,
pas de quoi se changer

« *t'as vu* »
… décourageants, les moindres soins de soi,
pour qui est plombé de fatigue et d'humidité, membre à membre,
en autant de poids insoulevables

contacts puants de la peau ou des muqueuses enflammées
à elles-mêmes,
boue et sécrétions les fondent ou soudent
aux plis et coutures des vêtements

se toucher écœure

*

quand il faisait trop froid,
il arrivait que des copains logés en foyer le fassent entrer en fraude dans la cuisine où dormir
quelques heures, tête sur la table (à cinq heures du matin, sortir…)
et dans l'aube attendre l'heure où s'ouvrirait, par exemple, la médiathèque où
(« on est gentil, personne dit rien »)
somnoler des heures…

*

Mais d'abord, il ne s'appelle pas « Ousmane ».

C'est lui qui, soudain, le **23 avril 2008** (alors que nous conversons depuis plusieurs mois), m'a demandé de ne pas écrire son « vrai nom » — celui qui figure, désormais, sur ses papiers.

Quel nom lui donner dans ce que j'écris ? lui ai-je demandé. Il m'a proposé celui d'un ami : Ousmane.
Ne serait-ce pas gênant, ou, qui sait, dangereux pour l'ami en question ?
Cet ami, m'apprend-il, est mort.

Ousmane a été tué en octobre 2003, dans le nord du Darfour, du côté d'El Fashir, alors qu'il cherchait à passer en Libye.
Personne, dit O., ne sait vraiment ce qui est arrivé. Tout le groupe avec lequel Ousmane voyageait, dans « un gros camion », a été tué. Les tueurs étaient sans doute des jenjawids, qui devaient savoir que ces voyageurs partaient pour la Libye, et qui ont voulu « l'argent des gens pour leurs passages » — et le camion.
Tout le monde est mort, répète O.

Mais la mort d'Ousmane, comment l'a-t-on sue ? Il avait une carte d'identité (lui qui avait vécu en ville) que la police a retrouvée.
Le responsable du village (« t'as vu, c'est pas exactement le maire, mais c'est un peu comme ça ») a été averti et a lui-même annoncé la mort d'Ousmane au village, à la famille : son père et sa mère, sa femme, ses deux enfants.

« Il avait 35-36 ans quand il est mort.
Il avait été mon ami pendant près de deux ans.
Il avait fait des études, il était intelligent. Il aurait pu trouver du travail.
Il avait travaillé à l'Est du Soudan, au bord de la mer Rouge, dans un port. Il s'était marié là.
Puis il avait emmené sa femme jusque dans l'Ouest du Soudan.
Au village, il habitait pas loin de chez moi. Pas la même famille, mais juste à côté. Mon grand-père connaissait sa famille. »

*

« Allez »... comment avancer enfin ?

Devrais-je reconstituer l'itinéraire d'O., et — au prix de recomposer ce qu'il m'en a dit (ne parlant presque jamais dans l'ordre chronologique, mais allant et revenant dans le temps) — faire s'en succéder les étapes réelles ?

Ou bien faudrait-il que la succession, ici, se réduise à être celle des notes que j'ai prises depuis des mois (avec, souvent, quelques heures, voire une nuit de décalage) d'après nos conversations ?

*

De quel début incontestable, ou du moins chronologiquement évident, aurais-je dû partir ? de juin-juillet 2007 ?

Ce fut alors, en réalité, un second début.
Dans une rue du centre de la ville, par hasard, un samedi soir, une nuit de fête (celle, je crois, de la musique), Hélène fut abordée par quelqu'un que d'abord elle ne reconnut pas mais qui — quoique difficile à comprendre (voix embarrassée, mots qui se cherchaient trop longuement au milieu des bruits ou sons éclatants dans la rue) — parvint à lui rappeler une rencontre de deux ans antérieure.
Il avait, par chance, un portable (cadeau ou prêt de copains) — dont il lui donna le numéro.

Le lendemain, un dimanche, donc, j'ai appelé. Ce n'est pas lui, mais un de ses amis — Hamid —, parlant assez bien le français, qui m'a répondu. Et nous avons pris un rendez-vous, eux deux, Hélène et moi, pour le lendemain : un lundi.

*

Mais ne faudrait-il pas que, d'abord, je remonte à la toute première rencontre (de deux ans plus ancienne) entre nous et O. ?
Et que je raccorde ce que j'écris ici — ou plutôt ce qu'à partir de notes je fixe (en juin 2008) — à ce que rapportaient des pages publiées il y a déjà plus d'un an dans *Po&sie* ?

Au bord de la Loire, un dimanche après-midi, en 2004, alertés par le correspondant du *Monde* à Orléans, nous avions rencontré des clandestins vivant dans de petits édicules en béton — probablement des abris de jardins ouvriers désaffectés — au milieu de broussailles.

Et puis nous avions, à leur demande, emmené deux d'entre eux d'abord à l'hôpital (en vain), puis chez un médecin de garde.

Ces deux-là, nous les avions enfin quittés dans les rues d'Orléans, non sans hésiter, au crépuscule.

Quelques jours plus tard, nous avions appris que la Préfecture avait fait transporter tous ces gens dans un centre d'hébergement provisoire, à quelque vingt ou trente kilomètres d'Orléans.
(Quant aux cabanes, elles avaient très vite été détruites, et le sol, débroussaillé, avait été livré aux promeneurs.)

O. était l'un des deux que nous avions accompagnés à une consultation médicale. Il avait été aussi, bien sûr, l'un de ceux que la Préfecture avait quelques jours plus tard fait héberger dans ce Centre où, pensions-nous, ils avaient pu, en tant que réfugiés du Darfour, attendre leur régularisation.

C'est donc après une longue interruption — un quasi-oubli, de notre côté, et pour O. la catastrophe du rejet par l'OFPRA — que la relation avec O. connut un second début.

*

Hier, 16 juillet 2007 — ai-je noté il y a bientôt un an —, fin d'après-midi, au Lutétia (face à la cathédrale — grand visage blanchâtre XVIIIe siècle ni vieux ni jeune, et soudain, le soir, se colorant d'orangé, face à l'ouest… illumination du ciel de Loire —, et non loin des blocs en dalles synthétiques des annexes administratives de la Préfecture),

quatrième rencontre avec O.
(après trois autres, où, urgence première, nous avions lu, Hélène et moi, les papiers qu'il transportait dans une chemise en carton verdâtre émiettée, et que seul son ami Hamid, lui aussi du Darfour, et qui était présent, avait pu, quelque peu, lui traduire).

C'était la première fois qu'O. venait seul. Hamid n'avait pu, cette fois, l'accompagner (un rendez-vous avec une assistante sociale).

Hamid qui, lors de nos trois précédentes rencontres à ce même Lutétia, jouait le rôle d'interprète n'a que vingt-deux ans. O. en a plus de trente.

Hamid a été à l'école jusqu'au niveau du bac, il a étudié l'anglais, il parle français, même si, dans un demi-sourire permanent, il parle trop bas, trop vite.
O. est — c'est du moins ce que je crois alors capter, mais j'apprendrai plus tard que son passé est plus compliqué — un paysan, il n'a fréquenté qu'un petit nombre d'années l'école coranique.

Lors de nos deux premières rencontres, O. ne nous a parlé que par l'intermédiaire de Hamid. Mais à la fin de la troisième rencontre — **9 juillet 2007** —, je me suis retrouvé seul avec lui, et j'ai constaté qu'il parlait — un français étrange, appris à écouter les jeunes dans les îles de la Loire, et, pour moi, à reconstituer, au vol…

C'est à l'issue de cette rencontre (la troisième) au café que j'ai emmené O. (à quelques centaines de mètres de là, près de la gare) chez Carrefour, pour lui acheter un sac de couchage et une petite tente (légère, dépliable d'un coup) (une petite chambre, a-t-il dit).

*

Ce qu'il a commencé à me dire de ses nuits dehors,
si, à tâtons, j'essayais d'en redire encore
quelque chose,
ce ne pourrait se faire sans incorporer ce que j'ai entendu vu ou imaginé autrement des mois plus tard, en le suivant sur les bords de la Loire, ce jour de novembre 2007 où nous sommes retournés sur des lieux (une maison vide squattée quelques jours en plein hiver) où ne subsistaient certes pas ses traces

mais où il m'en a montré d'autres,
à peu près semblables, disait-il,
pour lui, en tout cas, trop reconnaissables,
étrangères-familières
creux de couchage éphémère, nids d'herbes sales,
formes de corps, débris :
le très peu que laissent, en repartant le matin,
ceux qui doivent toujours tout emporter avec eux dans les rues
(couvertures, rares vêtements, un minimum d'aliments : rien ne peut être laissé sur
place — les employés municipaux ont instruction de tout ramasser ou détruire)

et chaque soir tout reformer
dans un minimum d'enroulement de soins de soi

*

et si c'était un enfant mien, adulte, déjà vieux, qui, par impossible, serait rencontré, épuisé, sans regard, au détour d'une rue étrangère (ou trop familière ?)

(terreur confondue dans la tendresse)

le temps s'est effondré devant lui il ne cesse de tomber dans un fossé plein de feuilles noires pourrissantes... (puanteur d'une tristesse absolue où se laisser submerger)

« ALLEZ VIENS » « tu vas pas rester là comme ça »... (et... impuissance se redouble — il ne désire plus rien — il n'est plus accessible)

« VIENS DONC »... impossible de l'arracher à cette décomposition de lui désormais trop connue, trop goûtée... « MAIS JE T'EN SUPPLIE VIENS... » « ALLEZ... »

*

Le 16 juillet (première conversation complètement seul à seul), sous le regard vaguement inquisiteur de la patronne du café (qui déjà nous reconnaît), j'ai interrogé O. sur sa vie au Darfour, avant que les violences — exercées par qui, au juste ? la question va courir dans ses propos ultérieurs — ne commencent ou, du moins, ne deviennent insupportables.

Il travaillait la terre, a-t-il dit, avec son père.
(Non, me suis-je dit plus tard en reprenant et entre-confrontant certaines de mes notes, son père, à l'époque, était mort. Et dans des conversations ultérieures, c'est de son grand-père qu'il parlera. Ou plutôt il aura d'abord dit : « grand-mère » puisque, m'expliquera-t-il, il parlait du père de sa mère.)

Ce qu'ils faisaient pousser, j'ai du mal à le comprendre. De la main, il me montre la hauteur des plantes.
On élevait des moutons. Il a insisté sur les agneaux, sur la possibilité de les vendre. Il a parlé du marché, et je n'ai pas bien compris ce qui pourtant paraissait important... un véhicule...

Soudain O. glisse — comme un rapide message en surplus, et en ajoutant que c'est la première fois qu'il le dit *(vais-je tout à l'heure, en rentrant chez moi, tirer de ces mots-là une satisfaction, celle d'inspirer confiance… nimbe rosâtre ému)* —
qu'il a songé à mourir.

Il parle encore des îles de la Loire, autrement que la fois précédente — d'une, particulièrement, qu'il aime bien. Belle, pour lui ? « Oui ».
Là, des gens viennent — des jeunes, des couples de jeunes — jusque tard dans la nuit, deux trois heures du matin… Gentils ? « Oui, oui » — « je les écoute ».

*

Après notre rendez-vous du 16 juillet, une chambre, un studio récemment aménagé (douche, WC, coin cuisine) et que nous louons, s'est trouvé libre au deuxième étage de notre maison (vaste vieille construction d'au moins deux siècles).
Nous avons pris la décision (qui restera active — dangereusement abstraite ? — dans toute la suite) de lui proposer d'habiter là.

Le 23 juillet, du Lutétia, où nous nous sommes retrouvés — de nouveau avec Hamid —, nous venons, traversant la Loire, à la maison. Je lui montre l'endroit. Il dit très vite, ou plutôt (visage baissé, larmes — d'humiliation ? — perlant) il fait dire par Hamid : « Je peux pas payer » (pendant que Hamid traduit, il fait un geste d'impuissance des deux mains), « même pas l'eau ou l'électricité ».

Silence où se fait soudain trop sensible, en connexions vitales, le plus banal.
Bruits dans les murs…
Trépidation douce des continuités-permanences, des connexions coûteusement partout entretenues : l'eau qui arrive (au bord de la Loire, la municipalité avait coupé l'eau…) ou les eaux (« usées » : évier, WC), qui s'évacuent, les câbles électriques (on en voit quelques-uns, lourds et noirs, par la fenêtre de ce second étage).

« Peux pas » — « Bien sûr ».

Silence. Cris de martinets ou, dans la lumière affluant horizontale du dehors, zébrure du vol d'une hirondelle s'engouffrant sous la gouttière proche…

« J'ai eu peur »… « Au fond du grand bateau, j'ai vomi, j'étais en sueur, j'ai cru que j'allais mourir »
Commencer par des phrases comme celles-ci, entendues des semaines plus tard ?

Un début au milieu de la Méditerranée (entre Libye et France), *in medias res*…
Du pathos ?
O. ne savait pas ce qu'était le mal de mer. « Si on me donnait une cigarette, elle me tombait de la bouche ». Il rit.

« J'ai pensé qu'on m'avait peut-être donné quelque chose avec la nourriture. Je n'osais plus manger. J'avais peur qu'on nous donne quelque chose et puis qu'on nous jette à la mer. »

« J'ai pensé que je reverrais jamais ma famille, ma mère, mes sœurs. Je pensais à mon grand-père. »

C'était en mai 2004, et la traversée a duré 8-9 jours : 2 jours sur un petit bateau (de pêcheur) (« en plastique » — est-ce bien ce qu'il a dit ?) et 7 jours sur le grand bateau.
Sur le petit bateau où il s'est trouvé, 7 personnes : 4 Soudanais, 2 Somaliens, 1 du Burkina Faso (le seul francophone).
Puis on se retrouve sur le grand bateau avec d'autres clandestins — 40 ? 50 ?

Sur le grand bateau, bien sûr, les clandestins ne sont pas tous ensemble. Ils sont cachés dans plusieurs endroits. Dans chacune des petites cabines destinées au repos du personnel, et prévues pour une ou deux personnes, on s'entasse à 7.
On a peur. On vous crie des choses qu'on ne comprend pas. On a peur que la police arrive : tout le monde alors irait en prison, même les gens qui travaillent sur le bateau.
Pas parler, pas tousser, pas éternuer.
(O. s'efforce de retrouver, de se souvenir de lui-même… Il sent bien que je cherche à m'approcher au plus près des sensations d'alors.)
« Lui il a peur », « moi j'ai peur », « c'est pas quelque chose normal ».
« On t'a pris le portable, la montre, le briquet, les papiers d'identité si tu en as, avant de monter dans le petit bateau : 'tu prends rien !' »

On mange une fois par jour.
Comment fait-on... pour pisser et pour... — c'est moi qui demande..., je suis un peu gêné — quels mots employer... Nos propos sont toujours retenus, pudiques. Gêné, mais pas trop, il rit : on pisse par un petit trou (un hublot ?). Et pour... le reste... dans du plastique... et tu jettes aussi par le trou.

Au moment d'arriver en France, en prenant un autre petit bateau, il a dû enfiler un uniforme de « la compagnie ».

Après débarquement, vers 21 h, on attend jusqu'à trois heures du matin. On boit un café. Un type nous prend en camion, nous emmène à la gare, paie le ticket jusqu'à Paris.
(Une autre fois, ou plutôt plusieurs fois, O. m'a expliqué le système compliqué de garantie avec les passeurs.)

Si j'ai bien compris, dans le train pour Paris, ils ne sont plus que deux.

*

À Paris, c'est le matin, on est là sur le trottoir, on connaît rien.

On voudrait un « petit service », un peu d'aide, un renseignement. On s'adresse, plusieurs fois, à des gens qui passent. On choisit toujours quelqu'un qui a l'air arabe, qui doit parler arabe. Mais toujours il se méfie, il a pas le temps, il sait pas.

Quelqu'un, encore, passe, parlant à son portable : en arabe. On essaie encore, on s'adresse à lui.
Il s'arrête.
Il écoute.

« & si c'est cela vivre ? »

À *« À ce qui n'en finit pas »*

« Non », dit Ousmane : **« c'est pas-ma-la-vie »**.

C'est au moins la deuxième fois que je transcris **ces mots** qu'Ousmane, Darfouri habitant chez nous depuis trois ans, a dits un jour, assis dans la cuisine :
ils **n'auront jamais fini,** ces mots-là, **de grelotter**… (même si ces derniers temps — mai 2010 — il m'arrive de sentir chez lui, sifflotant en repeignant en blanc, après l'avoir nappé d'enduit, un mur de la maison — des élans d'allégresse).

*

cette poignée de notes est prise d'une masse mouvante qui est et restera en cours

(plus qu'une succession, ces notes devraient former une ou des sphères de possibles pulsatiles)

*

Pour qui, et où, et quand, c'est… « pas une vie » ?

Il faut leur rendre **la vie impossible**, a dit un fonctionnaire de Préfecture — organisant, en effet, l'impossibilité glaciale et haineuse de tout soutien aux migrants, détruisant toute amorce d'une quelconque existence qui leur serait vivable.

*

« Auswandern » — émigrer — : titre d'un unique et incomparable (parmi ses œuvres) dessin de Klee daté de 1933.
Un couple fait de ratures dans du blanc, de rides dans un air plâtreux, d'incisions dans tout possible élément commun.

*

Vite ! c'est une guerre infime et sale.

Serait-ce ma guerre, attendue depuis toujours ? Ramasser en peu de phrases — sinon des vies, du moins des instants de l'« entre »-vies. **Condenser**, *rageusement… Que* **des instants** *(chair à vif) de vies intersectées se disent en* **projectiles** *…*
Contre quoi ?

*

Après une démarche pour essayer de sortir de l'impasse où restent bloqués les « papiers » d'Ousmane (établissement d'un « certificat de notoriété » chez un notaire) début 2010 ; nous (Ousmane, trois Français — les « témoins » soudanais ont repris en hâte le chemin de leur travail) allons boire un café au « Quick » non loin de la gare, dans le centre commercial (où je vais compulsivement tous les jours)… Chaleur (après le froid très vif du dehors, la neige gelée, etc.), vapeur des vêtements ou des corps. L'ami journaliste parle, inopinément, de conversations longues et intimes avec tel ami musulman — Afghan ? j'ai déjà oublié. « Il m'a expliqué, dit le journaliste, qu'il ne fallait pas parler de sa mère ». Ah oui ? Ousmane (brusquement joyeux — du fait, me dis-je, du soutien que nous nous sommes réunis pour lui apporter —, disert, dans son français où il a désormais beaucoup de vocabulaire, mais qu'il prononce mal en particulier du fait que — faute de se faire une représentation des phrases écrites ? — il segmente mal les mots, ne repère pas les articles, etc. — « l'équipe » (une de celles avec lesquelles il a travaillé en banlieue, par exemple, à couper des arbres dans la Loire) devient pour lui « les quipes » et ainsi naît un singulier privé de sa première syllabe, comme il arrive, il est vrai, à d'autres mots dans sa bouche) confirme : il en va également ainsi chez lui.
« Tu vois », dit-il (il me dit souvent, à la maison, « tu vois »), **« la mère, c'est comme un dieu »**.

Ai-je eu peur à cet instant ?

*

Le lendemain de la mort de ma mère (février 1996),
j'ai essayé, engourdi face à la baie vitrée
— nappes de perce-neige devinables avant le lever du jour
(mais comment formuler ce que deviennent, dans la nuit
leur blanc, leur vert, si naïvement crus — perçant comme de minuscules clous très aigus ?) —,
de « me dire » (obscur repli du soi à soi)
quelque chose.

Ai-je alors essayé de simplement « noter »
le semi-silence de cinq-six heures du matin ?

Grésillements ou coups externes-internes
se propageant,
sang dans les oreilles, échos dans les
murs, chaudière grondant derrière le mur,
ou, en enveloppes-pelures rose-sombre d'horizons auditifs,
voitures, roulements de poids
lourds ou de trains sur un pont sur
la Loire, avions parfois…

Soudain : brutalement (rêvée dans la somnolence gelée ?), une sonnerie
— appel ou injonction ?

Quel tracé de sang mental a sinué-perlé
griffant le temps plâtreux ?

Rien qu'un sifflement des narines noires-écailleuses du chien
qui, dans la cuisine, sur sa couverture sur le carrelage, avait dû s'enrouler, massif, et se serrait
contre lui-même en cherchant à se protéger du froid vif affluant sous la porte du jardin ou par les
interstices des fenêtres.

*

Est-ce que je voudrais — trop naïvement ? grossièrement ? — capter par instants et retenir
— ici par exemple, dans un minime réseau de phrases déjà grises —
ce qui fait l'envie de vivre ?
Cette brûlure réindéterminante qu'on se passe les uns aux autres (entre qui et qui ? à quels
instants précis ?) comme une chose qui n'existe qu'autant qu'elle glisse comme de main en
main ?

(Non…, c'était déjà, il y a un instant, dans les trois lignes qui précèdent, *trop dire*.)

*

Un jour de printemps 1995, chambre à « Sainte-Cécile »,
où — temps torpide —
ma mère survit.

Assise dans l'unique fauteuil (molesquine verte) où, incapable désormais
de marcher, elle passe des heures (jusqu'à ce qu'enfin quelqu'un la lève, la soulève),
semble endormie. Ses paupières
ne sont pas tout à fait closes : j'entrevois
par les minces fentes des yeux noyés.

Je regarde vaguement par la fenêtre rectangulaire (cadre métallique).
Rideaux de rayonne, fade odeur si familière,
de cela qui répond presque exactement aux prévisions
(sauf la poussière, ou la fatigue des matières
et l'affaissement des formes).

Me retournant vers elle : « je vais partir » lui dis-je.
« Je vais travailler »
(**Travailler ?** amère — comme en traces de doigts noirâtres de charbon sur la pâleur du passé — l'histoire de ce mot… entre nous).

Elle entr'ouvre les yeux : « Pourquoi ? », souffle-t-elle.
« Tu voudrais que je reste ? — Oui ! »
« Pourquoi ? » lui dis-je à mon tour, trop vite, presque méchamment
(avec l'impulsion de lui glisser, vainement, un : « À quoi bon ? »
ou : « Dans deux minutes tu auras oublié ! »).

De ses chuchotis égarés, j'ai alors entendu surgir, faible, un seul mot intelligible :
« **Personne** ».

*

Un autre jour *note d'avril 1991 sur laquelle*
je suis tombé hier soir 21 nov 09, en prenant et feuilletant au hasard un vieux cahier avant d'essayer de dormir,
ma mère n'étant pas encore dans une maison
de retraite (mon père l'avait déposée ici pour quelques
heures et on s'affairait en l'oubliant un peu), je l'ai entendue

— avec, sur le fond vert sombre du fauteuil, de petits
volètements de mains, puis, soudain, un index tendu —
marmonner (entre autres phrases folles et sombres, menaçantes) :
« **et il y en a qui mourront** ».

*

Ces notes... les dé-théâtraliser (les délivrer des inévitables minuscules poses et mises en scènes du soi notant) ?

Ou les déballer continûment de leurs protections contre ce dont (à travers tout « objet » momentané) elles parlent...

Et puis qu'elles ne subsistent que durement étalées : insectes écrasés sur quel mur ?

*

« *& si c'est cela vivre ?* »
Virginia Woolf, *Journal*, 25 nov 1928
« [...] Ainsi passent les jours et je me demande quelquefois si nous ne sommes pas hypnotisés par la vie comme l'est un enfant par une boule d'argent ? *& si c'est cela vivre ?* C'est très rapide, brillant, excitant, mais peut-être aussi superficiel. J'aimerais prendre la boule dans mes mains ; la palper doucement, ronde, lisse et lourde, *&* la tenir ainsi, jour après jour. Je vais lire Proust je crois, et revenir en arrière, puis repartir en avant. »

*

29 juillet 2007 20h45 — À travers la vieille baie vitrée sont visibles des entrecroisements de branches, tiges, feuilles : ils ruissellent de pluie, plus ou moins loin, et diversement éclairés (avec des nuances de vert-brun, de mauve ou violet) par le jour qui baisse.
Ce hasard des végétaux et de leurs croissances respectives (ou celui de mon regard, de ma position)
— tout est soudain si juste, à la dérobée, vibrant,
accordé.
Elle brûle, dans l'air tendrement acide (Pérugin), **cette musicalité arbitraire,** toujours neuve : elle est — plus qu'elle ne le fut jamais pour des humains, dans « notre » *mais, nez contre la vitre, ce « nous », dans ce que je « me » dis, m'étouffe comme du biscuit fade*

acosmisme —
une surprise
incompréhensible.

*

1949-1950 ? Quelque dimanche soir… :
Vitres peintes en bleu (contre ce qui avait été *juin 44* attaques aériennes en pleine nuit)…
demeurées longtemps comme aveuglées, éblouies par la lumière du soir.
Odeurs — troublant le temps — de couleurs, souffles de silhouettes en ciment écorché,
ou en métal noir et par places rouillé.
Se découpent, dans la hâte de rentrer à la maison, sur le ciel orangé,
un château d'eau, un gazomètre…

*Graffiti — apparus sur quel support ? — d'une dévorante séduction infantile : l'éblouissement de
la guerre.*

*

et du jaune velouté : les flancs irrégulièrement arrondis voire
grumeleux de quelques coings encore sur l'arbre

**… sensations (nov 09) dont aucune n'est vitale ni nécessaire mais qui, à travers leurs
hasards, donnent ce dont il est terrible d'être (et spécialement par la haine organisée)
privé…**

*

« une merveille infiniment chère et douce »
(une merveille à faire surgir en décrivant rien qu'allusivement ?)
Leopardi, *Zibaldone* (8 ?), j'ai noté ce passage dans un
cahier de 91-92 il y a donc (aujourd'hui, en 2009) au moins
dix-sept ans, et, sottement, sans autre identification…
« … Décrivant en peu de touches, ne montrant que peu de chose de l'objet, [les Anciens]
laissaient l'imagination errer dans le vague et l'indéterminé de ces idées enfantines qui
naissent de l'ignorance du tout. Et une scène champêtre, par exemple, peinte par un poète

antique en quelques traits et, pour ainsi dire, sans horizon, suscitait dans l'imagination ce céleste ondoiement d'idées floues et brillantes, d'un romanesque indéfinissable et d'une étrangeté, d'une merveille infiniment chère et douce, semblable à celle qui faisait les extases de notre enfance. »

*

Reçue, l'adhésion à la vie — même si elle prend l'allure d'une simple et minimale apparence d'auto-approbation, même si elle n'est qu'un négligeable redoublement
comme un ressaut vif-figé de pierre truitée sous de l'eau courante
qui se sera formé jadis et qui doit se recréer, s'il se peut, tout au long d'une existence.

Cette adhésion s'est engendrée et se réalimente **dans la si fruste certitude qu'on fut** et peut-être qu'on est encore *fût-ce en dormant, joue contre quelque appui* soutenu dans la vie et porté, dans la clarté, comme par une paume,
désiré, oui — d'où ? par qui ou quoi ? —, être en vie.

*

De plusieurs femmes qui, à peine adolescentes, furent déportées (Anne-Lise Stern ?), je crois avoir lu ou entendu qu'elles eurent la certitude (avec confiance ? avec douleur ?) d'avoir à **rapporter quelque chose à leur mère : leur vie.**

*

« **Quelque chose de blanc, d'infiniment blanc** » : couleur de la terreur ? de la mort de tout lien, de la plus élémentaire confiance ?
Je n'ai pas, me dis-je, la place, ici, de recopier un poème de Ritsos, qu'on ne peut lire sans ravage : un de ses poèmes de détention dans des camps. Il dit, s'infiltrant entre les prisonniers, **la perte de la confiance la plus élémentaire … Et c'est un pâlissement de tout**
Le poème a d'abord dit comment l'un d'eux parut désirer parler :

> *[…] Personne*
> *ne le croit plus ; ne le regarde plus — qu'il dise ce qu'il veut.*

Mais quand le poème en vient à former-formuler le non-rapport, c'est dans l'invention la plus précise, en images qui se moulent, avec une cruelle exactitude, sur l'impossibilité (« **masque de verre** » !)

> *Non que nous ayons eu peur de cet apeuré — pas du tout. Une vitre*
> *plus haut, du cinquième étage, jetait sur lui une douce lueur ;*
> *lui éclairait le visage comme s'il portait un masque de verre.*
> *Et nous*
>
> *alors nous portions les mains au visage comme pour nous cacher*
> *ou comme pour soutenir un mur qui penche. Entre nos doigts*
> *tombaient des morceaux de plâtre, des pierres, de la poussière, des pièces cuivrées ;*
> *nous nous baissions et les ramassions ; sans nous agenouiller devant lui.*

Alors vient le « blanc » : un calme affreux ?

> *Et dans le miroir, en face, quelque chose de blanc, d'infiniment blanc —*
> *un vieux peigne en os dans un verre d'eau,*
> *et la lumière sereine de l'eau dans le verre, dans le miroir, dans l'air.*
> *Yaros, 24.05.68*

*

Ousmane me parle de son grand-père maternel (celui qui, après la mort du père à Nyala, avait accueilli la famille à la campagne, celui aussi — autres bribes de récits dans la cuisine — qui parlait avec la mère dans une langue qu'Ousmane ne comprenait pas, ce grand-père, enfin, qui mourut peu après la fuite d'Ousmane… *d'où l'angoisse d'avoir laissé des femmes seules exposées à… quoi ?*)
et ce qui vient dans ses propos lents *du temps, à la faveur des difficultés linguistiques, s'introduisant dans ses pensées*, c'est une présence souvent silencieuse — mais qui parfois racontait des décennies anciennes, des parcours à travers l'Afrique.

*

Ousmane, lui ai-je demandé un jour, **qu'est-ce qui est beau pour toi ?**
(C'était avant qu'il repeigne ici avec presque des méditations préalables, avec tant de goût : nuances, plusieurs blancs, et de l'ocre pâle…)

« C'est quand j'ai fait une chose, en bois, en terre, qui peut rester là dans la maison, et qu'on peut voir plusieurs fois, chacun, ma mère, mes sœurs... »

*

Sortir dans le jardin — **dans une aube de mai** pleine de brume.
Vieille petite utopie d'**une attention-bientôt-écriture lilliputienne : se ramifier** dans le tout connu *en rigoles de curiosité enfantine mi-sexuelle parmi de tendres chairs végétales, brillantes, perlant...*
afin de mieux guider, dans tous les rapports, replis, éboulis, des cohortes de petits insectes noirs identifiables mais toujours surprenants,
afin d'insinuer des mots — pour... disparaître
absorbé (comme s'il allait se refermer, lèvre contre lèvre, tel qu'on pourrait enfin n'avoir jamais été)
par le réel

*

**Depuis le seuil d'une maison crûment éclairée au-dedans, quelqu'un
crie**

crie à qui ?

à un(e) enfant partant à vélo (phare de travers sur le garde-boue *un halo ocre-rose va se mettre à tressauter sur le gravier luisant d'une route apparaissant à mesure* cliquetis de chaîne qui déjà se fond dans le bruit d'une pluie noire battante)

crie, d'une voix de colère :
« Au moins, rentre vivant(e) ! »

Aube perpétuelle ?

…les heures de la nuit d'avant le jour, les étirer… et qu'elles craquèlent en fissures blanches — perlant alors de possibles notes, de micro-libertés (qui vont s'évaporer)…

*

Des ébauches — mais en quoi impossibles à *réellement* reprendre ?

*

Il n'y a pas de mots, quand le jour se lève, en mars, **pour l'évidence** de la fraîcheur **du ciel** ou **pour sa matière** (presque une chair) la plus réelle — et donc introuvable

c'est une chance

ou de l'irréfutable

entre les arbres échelonnés
dans l'air rouge

cerisiers nus (des bandes d'écorce se sont enroulées pendant l'hiver, gouttelettes de suc orange), ou branches s'élevant au-dessus, tout au fond, théâtrales et poudrées, du cèdre…

*

Notes de pré-aube : en elles, quel dur *de fait* ?

les écrire — les « fixer » —, **c'est les retrouver telles qu'elles** n'ont jamais existé,
et cependant comme déjà là,
telles qu'elles **se sont** (graffiti virtuels dans le sommeil, ou entre moments et états dénivelés de la journée, ou dans la rue, ou en s'occupant de tout autre chose, etc.)
précédées elles-mêmes.

*

Matériaux, encore en attente, un certain nombre de **ces notes ?**
à « reprendre » un jour ?

quel geste faudrait-il alors, quel rabattement quasi transcendant (comme un pli voûté de lourde étoffe bleue brune), ou quel retournement d'une main soudain libre dans une inaccessible quatrième dimension ?

(aujourd'hui, ici, rien ne glisse sur ces phrases ébauchées sinon — les réduisant à ce qu'elles sont — une lame.)

*

Voici qu'en s'astreignant à se fixer ici ces notes (comme se cherchant réciproquement, se palpant l'une l'autre de phrases-antennes) tendent à se lier : **tentation de narrativité**, ici, ou, là, **tentative d'interrogation plus continue** …

Renoncent-elles alors à leur autonomie, à leurs multiples micro-libertés ?

*

Mais aussi : par certaines notes — comme celles-ci —, y aurait-il à délivrer, à déverrouiller et **déclencher, une** plus mordante et broyante **activité** (comme de mandibules chitineuses, noires orangées, d'insectes constamment au travail)
susceptible de devenir celle, quasi insue,
de notes futures ?

de leur minime activité perpétuelle ces notes à venir attaqueraient

elles sauraient s'en prendre directement aux tenues des choses réelles

s'agrippant aux emprises vitales transperçant les consistances-croyances
elles en feraient s'exprimer les sucs vitaux-rêvés

*

Ce fut souvent, des années durant, sous l'effet et par l'effort d'autres tentatives se consacrant à des « sujets » déterminés (avec une obstination comme butée *ainsi ma récente — mais vieille de combien d'années ? — tentative sur la puissance de la bêtise*),
qu'auront suinté certaines notes…

surcroît, alors, bleu de prusse,
sueur qui perle…

Et pourtant c'est celles-là mêmes qui seront restées en connivence avec l'indolence ordinaire ; elles n'ont pas cessé d'incorporer du temps sans but, le plus vitalement fade.

*

À l'aube, mais si tard, reviennent (pour n'avoir jamais été notées ?) — comme des odeurs, des chuchotis ou des parasitages de l'immédiat — **de marmonnantes « sensations politiques »**…

…constitutive fut, dans les années d'immédiate après-guerre (deuxième guerre mondiale),
contre la joue,
l'odeur-souffle d'un poste de radio, chaude :
bakélite et poussière, elle émanait d'une petite demeure derrière un rectangle de toile verdâtre tendue (auprès de la petite vitre portant les noms des stations) ;
une minuscule ampoule, filaments orangés, y brûlait

des voix, peut-être des micro-personnages logés là, tressautaient bougeaient…

voix nasillardes dans la cuisine mesquine d'alors : elles venaient du fond de l'espace comme aujourd'hui de celui du passé

aride, ce fut bientôt le temps de la guerre de Corée, 1950-53 (« Temps du monde : la Corée » écrivit à l'époque Vittorio Sereni),
il s'insinuait comme une odeur en trop dans celles de l'entre-soi familial

*

…et l'Indochine ? l'Algérie ? énormes masses, pressions inflexions courbures orangées de tout le passé

les faire venir... dans quelle attention d'après-coup,
les dilater nuages-terres sanglants

les dilacérer enfin, rageusement, dans un coin, suppléant l'enfant qui ne pouvait...

*

ah! (8 h, début mars) : qu'est-ce qui vient de cligner dans la minute précédente, au-dehors ?

aux ramifications noires qui sur fond du ciel pâle de l'aube paraissent, vues d'ici (à travers les vieilles vitres, verruqueuses par endroits), aussi fines
que des mailles

s'est pris... quoi... une palpitation — **un battement**, probablement, d'aile (à contre-jour),
ramier ou corneille...

et tout le senti a été, vibrant comme une toile,
brièvement sûr

rien de « nécessaire »... mais... si cela
n'arrivait plus
jamais... alors... quelle
mort ?

*

C'est tout simplement qu'elles sont infixables, ces notes : dès qu'elles se saisissent, si peu que ce soit, de ce qu'elles désirent, elles perdent toute stabilité.

*

Une vie durant : de la « poésie-peut-être » ?

bien sûr, pas de nom pour ça, jadis, dans l'enfance, après-guerre (en rentrant le soir, dans la rue grise orangée... décombres blancs béants)

impossible, en ce temps-là, d'en parler ou de s'en rien dire...

poésie, cependant, **comme arrachement ?**

espoir de jadis… à reconnaître enfin ?

avoir prise
en certains instants (dans les odeurs d'herbes agrippantes au pied des murs), par la seule faiblesse-force du sentir
sur quelles puissances mouvantes qui
se retournant sur « moi » — *sur la charge qu'il se révélait impossible de ne pas être pour soi-même*
m'auraient arraché de ma place,
ou auraient ressaisi ma propre réalité
— pour la refondre et
me faire substantiellement devenir ce qui ne serait plus, enfin,
un « soi » que mêlé de souffles libres, d'éclaircies, d'altérités palpitantes…

*

Rien, dans ces notes, ne se sera réellement mis en mouvement si elles ne se simultanéisent pas sensiblement (dans quels éclairs d'évidence ?)
avec
ce qu'il doit en être pour les autres
— c'est-à-dire encore pour moi (la question me revenant plus vive d'être passée « au-dehors ») —
du désir ou de l'espoir, vague peut-être mais tenace, de « se restituer »…

Que puis-je en savoir, en percevoir, en deviner, dans la rue par exemple ? Quoi d'autre que de pauvres idées, de grossières représentations (il n'y aurait, chez « les gens », que résignation à de l'effondrement lent, ou une décomposition vague du « soi »… — mais non… peut-être pas…) ?

*

Politiques, certaines au moins — depuis toujours — des sensations ? N'auront-elles pas plutôt été des résistances ou objections à toute politique (effective ou possible) ?

Moussant rageuses dans le plus familier, souvent impuissantes, ces sensations… : rebelles ? « petites bourgeoises » ?
Non non… je défigure bêtement… comment retracer ce qui là se refuse et fuit ?

NOTES

*

Réalisme brusque (au réveil) des liens ou liaisons et connexions :

une douche dans la nuit (fouillis de branches de glycine vaguement éclairées par le vasistas) (gel dehors ?) :
l'eau chaude dans le bruit du chauffe-eau, sa chaleur je la sens soudain comme soustraite à quoi ?
et puis tout, brusquement, l'eau, le gaz, les fils électriques, se rappelle comme ce que c'est : aboutchements, prises sur des forces, des réalités ailleurs préparées, du temps soutiré, une sorte de suc circulant s'échappant et…

dégoût, soudain, de cette sensation multi-ombilicale
dans la vapeur ?
dangereuse la tentaculaire dépendance ainsi réalisée *tout pourra toujours — voire voudra — s'éteindre ou se tarir*

*

« **What do we depend on to make us feel alive, or real ?** Where does our sense come from, when we have it, that our lives are worth living ? »
Adam Phillips (qui cite Winnicott : « If you show me a baby you certainly show me also someone caring for a baby, or at least a pram with someone's eyes and ears glued to it. One sees a 'nursing couple'. »)

Dépendances, oui, à jamais ? Consubstantialités de vies… (Henry Moore : liens réalisés — en bronze).

*

Se défaire, enfin… de quoi ? Se faire plus que nu ?

Hwang Ji-u : « Quand j'enlève mes vêtements dans la salle de bains, il y a quelque chose d'autre que j'aimerais enlever. »

*

Une doublure-attention continue et indéchirable pour tout ce qui pourrait arriver... :
ces notes seraient-elles autant de traces morcelées de la recherche d'une réalisation à quoi
en général on renonce (se contentant de rêveries diurnes) ?

Du « mien » ou du tout autre, vibrant au fil des minutes ? ...

Une altérité translucide s'étirant pour chacun tout le long du jour, se moulant sur les
événements de toute espèce, **collée en une tunique contre les moindres instants**, et les
consumant à mesure...

*Utopie intime... sourdant, par moments, irrépressible, pour chacun ? — dans la fatigue de la rue,
dans le train ou au fil des occupations obligatoires...*

de l'inévitable chez quiconque
et, simplement, s'exposant dans les présentes notes ?

*

Ou des notes, vite, au moins virtuelles, vivement abouchées aux coupures, aux
intersections du temps

et surtout buvant
entre sommeil / rêve et
réveil

: il faut qu'elles dérivent leur vie là
où les attentes ou doutes de la veille, se réouvrant
(dans la brusquerie des gestes pour se rhabiller..., luttant avec les tubes ou embranchements
à odeurs que sont les vêtements...),
ne peuvent,
vaisseaux tranchés dans l'air,
que sangloter de la substance psychique

*

Des fourmillements soudain réapparaissent, dans la lumière d'aube, ou sous le néon de
la cuisine, et grouillent (alors que je croyais avoir fixé quelques phrases : ce peu de notes)

micro-terreur…
plus que n'importe quelles autres, les phrases des « notes » devraient ne jamais faire oublier celles, à demi formées, multiples, fuyantes, contradictoires, qui les ont précédées…

Tout achèvement unifiant-broyant donnerait-il à ces notes un goût de mensonge…, une odeur d'insectes écrasés ?

*

Renaissent-elles toujours, ces notes
…proliférantes ébauches comme une végétation d'emblée sèche ?

pour se dérober, à toute puissance d'un tout en formation et qui exigerait que chaque esquisse locale se donne à l'ensemble, se sacrifie ou, du moins, se laisse précisément contenir par ce qui lui mesurerait sa place…?

Cette instance d'un « tout » : l'œuvre au sens « absolu » de Flaubert — et « reçue » par Kafka — se trouverait-elle tacitement confrontée à l'appartenance sociale au sens moderne, à l'état-nation et (projetée massivement par exemple dans Salammbô) à sa monstruosité sacrificielle ?

(Qu'est-ce qui peut en être sensible dans les dérobements constants de ces notes ?)

*

Et cette autre prolifération, celle des paroles dans la conversation ?

Porc, me suis-je dit en me voyant (m'étant arraché un instant, presque malgré moi, à la conversation à l'étage au-dessus) dans la glace sale au-dessus du lavabo des toilettes du café, tu es rosâtre d'excitation verbale.

Qu'est-ce qui m'a pris ? pourquoi cette volubilité démentant instantanément tout ce à quoi j'aurais voulu croire tenir ?

Cette excitation (chaleurs des joues) se retrouve-t-elle dans mes notes ? *me suis-je demandé, écœuré, dans le train, la rue, la nuit, au-dessus de la Loire.*

*

« Plus que tout j'écarterais ces paroles que les lèvres plutôt que l'esprit choisissent, ces paroles pleines d'humour, comme on en dit dans la conversation, et qu'après une longue conversation avec les autres on continue à s'adresser facticement à soi-même et qui nous remplissent l'esprit de mensonges, ces paroles toutes physiques qu'accompagne chez l'écrivain qui s'abaisse à les transcrire le petit sourire, la petite grimace qui altère à tout moment, par exemple, la phrase parlée de Sainte-Beuve, tandis que les vrais livres doivent être les enfants non du grand jour et de la causerie mais de l'obscurité et du silence. » Proust, *Recherche*)

*

Le bavardage intérieur : inévitable — ou même quasi corporel, et moussant, vital ?

alors… se découvrir continûment en train de secréter un flot de quasi-mots ? est-ce le matériau nécessaire pour tout ce qu'on peut tenter de penser/dire ? comment s'allier, formant des phrases, à cette production crépitante ?

*

Qu'est-ce qui, avant toute parole (ou après elle, la ravalant),
bouillonne et clapote **« dans la tête » de chacun** *au milieu même de la rue*

quelles ébauches de phrase anticipées, mal formées, se refondant, cuisant…
pour laisser place soudain à ce qui, irrémédiablement, se trouve dit

*

…d'un poème (auto)railleur de Zbigniew Herbert : « **La voix intérieure** »…

(cette sorte d'existence mythique du dedans… dont on ne sait ce qu'elle est avant qu'on parle et se fasse entendre des autres ou de soi comme autre,
cette présence plus réelle que tout, et néanmoins constamment virtuelle…)

« […] elle est peu audible / presque inarticulée // même en se penchant très profond / on n'entend que des syllabes / dénuées de sens […] // parfois même / j'essaie de lui parler / — tu sais hier j'ai refusé / je n'ai jamais fait cela / je ne vais pas commencer // — glou — glou // — alors tu crois

/ que j'ai bien fait // — gua — guo — gui // c'est bien qu'on soit d'accord // — ma — a // — repose-toi maintenant / nous reparlerons demain // elle ne me sert à rien / je pourrais l'oublier [...] »

*

La justesse : ne saurait-elle venir qu'après de la prolifération d'abord vaine ou plus ou moins grotesque ?
Faut-il qu'elle soit appelée, et rendue douloureusement nécessaire, par des phrases d'abord étouffées-étouffantes... et à... guérir ?

*

Quand vient-il opportunément, ici (ou quand viendrait-il, s'il venait), **le moment de fixer des phrases : d'un féroce regard-écoute,** s'abattre sur du trop abondant

se recourber, fouiller du bec, dilacérer...
aérer de vides perçants...

... trouver le rythme en un *second temps* ?

*

Comme induite par des ébauches trop épaisses (soupe verdâtre),
il arrive soudain — il faut ? — que s'insinue et que rage, seconde,
une spatialisation intense
(animée de quelles forces ?)

... de l'espacement, oui, alors, des souffles, du jugement tacite-tactile, des déroulements qui se libèrent brusquement, ou de l'en même temps qui s'impose non unifiable,

(se crée-t-il alors
— comme sous les pesées de pas qui se poseraient / lèveraient, trouvant le blanc de brun-mauve —
des places, des possibilités de « compter »... ?)

*

... quoi, alors, d'analogue à de ... la « loi » (au sens Lefort) ?

une force-souffle d'espacement ou de soulèvement de toutes les positions de mots dans une phrase ou un vers

analogue (non, davantage : c'est sans doute le même élan) aux positions-poids des vies dans l'« entre » ?

chacun se révélant n'être soi que par le passage de l'être-soi en qui que ce soit, indéfiniment

*

« lois brûlées dans l'éclair du calme » (Nelly Sachs)

*

À reconnaître aussi, dans ces notes, des matériaux possibles (pour un temps qui ne viendra que douteusement ?)...

des tas de terre mentale, des amas de confusion, des chantiers abandonnés sous quel vent de panique (fuite...)
et restés à béer sous la pluie
dans l'air blanc... ?

*

Parfois, encore et encore, furieusement, s'acharner sur le déjà fait, sur le trop formé-formulé — et le redécomposer en micro-entités s'évadant, se perdant dans le brouillard ?

*

Revenir (en retraversant parfois des années, parfois quelques jours ou simplement deux ou trois heures) **sur ce que, en général, j'ai écrit, serait-ce me couler contre mon propre cadavre ?**

Peau encore vivante contre peau glacée pas tout à fait morte... Sueur froide dans l'entre corps, dans le contact mi-vie/mi-mort...

... devant le poste de garde d'une cour de caserne (en Lorraine),
en pleine nuit, dans cette camionnette de la gendarmerie où je n'avais pu entrer qu'en rampant à tâtons,
c'est d'un coup,
et de tout mon propre corps,
que je découvris que ce jeune soldat (vingt ans comme moi)
dont on venait de me dire qu'il était blessé et attendait des soins
était en réalité déjà froid

alors il fallut ...

Tout seul, Khaled ?

mars 2015 — août 2015

« je veux pas rester tout seul » a dit Khaled

ces paroles-là, je ne finirai jamais de les réentendre… et la voix, sourde, granuleuse, combien familière
plus que proche aujourd'hui même
— malgré

*

ne pas être seul, mais être perdu,
c'est comme si sa propre douleur et celle d'un autre
enfantaient un troisième cœur

Vladimir Holan, *En marche*

*

rien qu'une amorce, ces lignes, dans le désarroi :
du trop tôt trop tard
rien, ici aujourd'hui, qu'un
« pour qu'il soit dit »

*

aujourd'hui ?

dans le temps — jour après jour, d'heure en heure — des masses de migrants
fuyant « chez nous »
l'invivable régnant « chez eux » (ces enfers de l'expansion desquels
« nous » aurons été,
aveugles ou cyniques,
partie prenante)

NOTES

informations du **29 juillet 2015**, France Musique 7 heures…
migrants qui cherchent à passer à Calais vers l'Angleterre

> Khaled aussi avait fait, en 2006 je crois, une tentative
> — il ne me l'avoua que
> tardivement et allusivement
> …par honte ? regret ?

ou, au hasard, Mediapart : au lendemain du naufrage survenu **le mercredi 5 août**
au large des côtes libyennes, les garde-côtes italiens annoncent 370 rescapés…
le bateau qui transportait au moins 600 migrants a chaviré, puis coulé.

À quoi bon insérer là ces deux informations presque instantanément caduques là où
pourraient-devraient chaque jour se déverser des centaines et milliers d'autres images

> *visions disponibles de radeaux de la Méduse en plastique se dégonflant*
> *(l'autre jour chez un ami soudanais dans un* HLM *de la banlieue*
> *d'Orléans dans une brève vidéo sur un téléphone portable qu'on me tendait*
> *j'entendais vrombir un invisible hélicoptère alors qu'une forme orange*
> *basculait sur-dans la mer, que des têtes étaient visibles : surnageant,*
> *disparaissant)*

> (non) comptages de corps disparus

> alors **notre « entre nous »,**
> **celui des vies qui se croient ordinaires,**
> **s'envenime, œdématisé,**
> **cyanosé**

*

« dans » cet ordinateur, donc, auront attendu, attendent encore — en vain ? —
des milliers de notes — quasi immédiates, factuelles, s'il se peut, jusqu'à la brutalité — d'un
« *Avec Khaled* »

traces disparates et répétitives, amassées huit années durant et qu' « il faudrait » reprendre pauvres,
sèches terreuses
quasi organiques : sales

*

>   *mais n'est-ce pas d'abord*
>   **les choses mêmes à noter**
>   *qui s'étaient amassées sans fin*
>
>   bouts de conversations sans nombre
>   évidences qui clignèrent une minute
>   peurs-colères rires questions sans réponses
>   clartés et doutes

*

ramasser tout cela dans les mois qui viennent, le relever,
le surélever,
le faire tenir par soi-même
— en quel tombeau ?

une voûte à la Kleist (celle qu'il dit dans une lettre à Wilhelmine) :
ne tenant en l'air que par le désir de toutes ses pierres de tomber

*

>   *Toi, mon ami ! ô comme j'ai tremblé du froid de ce*
>   *poème,*
>   *j'avais si peur des mots que je biaisais encore.*
>   *Je commençais des vers … Je m'efforçais d'écrire à*
>   *propos d'autre chose,*
>   *en vain, et la nuit, cette terrible nuit qui s'embusque*
>   *me commande :*
>   *C'est de lui qu'il faut parler !*
>
>   Miklos Radnoti, Cinquième Églogue

*

« pas tout seul »

c'était le 15 mars 2015 *un peu avant 11 h*
il venait de descendre de sa chambre
il était, contre toute habitude, hésitant — regard tourné au-dedans

il s'est assis dans le vieux fauteuil vert
face à moi
j'ai essayé comme si souvent de le faire rire

mais déjà sans doute
il ne m'entendait plus

il a dit ça

*

ces paroles, Khaled n'aura pas eu la force d'avoir peur à l'instant où il les a prononcées…

mais moi n'aurais-je pas dû sur-le-champ (ce fut il est vrai une affaire de minutes)
deviner
la catastrophe qu'elles annonçaient ?

il était là dans le fauteuil vert et j'ai eu peur qu'il ait froid (ce matin de printemps était gris et glacial)

je l'ai reconduit à sa chambre (qu'en général — radiateur électrique réglable — il surchauffait), j'ai préparé une tisane, lui ai tendu la tasse

et

*

*ne suis-je pas en train, parlant de lui, de ce « nous » hésitant que nous fûmes,
de me parer de l'oripeau infect et vaniteux
du deuil ?*

*

Je préférerais ne plus penser si ça doit aussitôt se traduire comme ça. Il est des pensées, Julie, pour lesquelles il ne devrait pas exister d'oreilles. Ce n'est pas bien, qu'elles crient à la naissance, comme des enfants.

Büchner, *La mort de Danton*

*

ramassant — pour les former-formuler —
quelques poignées de notes des instants de la mort de Khaled

je ne peux bien sûr éviter d'imaginer pour elles
quelque accueil possible
mais c'est aussitôt
plus follement que jamais
avec
rage et répulsion

sang de ronces qui rouillent
la revoilà (du fond de l'enfance)
la plus que connue
l'archaïque saveur

le venin
d'un délire :

les phrases ici
vont
se remettre à se tordre

elles s'acharnent à réaliser
le désir d'être délivré
du désir d'être reçu

*

Khaled Mahjoub Mansour, l'ami soudanais, le dimanche 15 mars un peu après 11 heures a été abattu devant moi par un infarctus

deux heures durant on essaya de relancer les palpitations du cœur

il est resté près de trois jours en salle de réanimation à l'hôpital de La Source (au sud d'Orléans)
il est mort le 18 mars 2015, un peu après 23 heures

*

NOTES

le samedi 14 mars, il était revenu de près de deux mois passés au Soudan
un séjour au cours duquel il avait dû, pour des raisons familiales, accomplir un voyage épuisant
c'est ce qu'il avait commencé à raconter dans notre conversation brève (il était épuisé) de ce samedi soir
en camion (pour économiser le coût de l'avion)
de Khartoum à Nyala

sa ville natale, au Darfour

il m'avait raconté, par bribes, les marchés où
des années plus tôt,
enfant il allait vendre je ne sais quoi avec son père

petit véhicule…, petits voyages
et à l'heure de midi, lové dans l'ombre sous l'étal,
joie minuscule d'un « p'tit cadeau » : un « p'tit gâteau »

un interminable trajet coupé par une longue interruption (du fait d'obscures escarmouches)
trois ou quatre jours, donc, dans l'extrême chaleur… parfois sans eau
etc.

*

samedi 14 mars, vers 15 heures, après des semaines d'absence (trop rares, ses appels à partir d'un portable… *depuis des régions souvent sans réseau m'avait-il expliqué en hâte lors d'une de nos communications*)

c'est de France qu'enfin il avait appelé
il était gare du Nord

« allo allo » — avais-je entendu (reconnaissant aussitôt sa voix)
puis un rire familier
puis
« allo allo c'est le connard Mansour »

tel était notre mot de passe
la plus minable de nos plaisanteries ritualisées
au goût de vieille chaussure

« canards et connards »
deux canards de Loire dérivaient le long de la rive
où marchaient deux hommes,
réglant sur eux la vitesse de leur marche

nous deux allant
à la recherche des endroits où K. avait naguère dormi
(certains mois par des nuits glaciales à l'aube desquelles
il lui était arrivé, m'avait-il dit, de songer au suicide),

« deux connards regardent deux canards,
deux canards regardent deux connards »
n'est-ce pas en janvier 2008, que je les lui avais dits, ces mots imbéciles ?

cette trouvaille, stupide bien sûr, auto-réalisatrice ici même,
il l'avait aussitôt adoptée avec un rire sardonique

*

vital, le rire entre nous — ou comme en deçà de nous…
(ce que je lui disais pour le faire rire, ne le recevais-je pas de lui ?)

rire infra-quoi ? infra toi-moi

nous riions du fait d'être quelqu'un
de la nécessité d'avoir, chacun ensemble,
à être quelqu'un

*

canard ou connard…
et un hasard :
je viens de tomber fin juillet 2015 sur
la « Préface — Résultante » de
La Gueule de Rechange (dans La Chair et l'Idée)
*de **Sony Labou Tansi***

Quelle est mon Dieu cette idée qui vaut la peine qu'on crève avec ? Celle-ci peut-être : « La bourgeoisie est tellement sale que le communisme devient enfantin. » Or il faut choisir, à tout prix. Et mon choix le voici : Ni sale, ni enfant.

Et si j'ai choisi, comprenez que ce n'est pas ma faute, c'est la faute de mon siècle. Tous ceux qui choisiront avec moi sont « conaristes » bien entendu, mais ils auront la paix. La paix du conard, différente fort heureusement de la paix du canard. Et puis, ils ne seront pas si cons que ça, puisqu'ils auront prévu quelque chose pour demain, là où le communisme ne prévoit qu'un soir et la bourgeoisie sa propre chute.

SLT

*

de l'avoir à être soi, aurai-je encore et encore voulu croire

dès le temps du lycée
(années obscures — 1956 ou suivantes : Hongrie, Algérie)

conférences
— pour des poignées d'auditeurs dans une salle minuscule d'Orléans —

contre la guerre d'Algérie,
ou sur l'Afrique du Sud — un film documentaire tourné clandestinement dans des mines, avec soudain le chant de
Miriam Makeba —

… ou bien, entendues dans la quasi obscurité
— lumignon d'un obscur conférencier —
des pages de
Michaux, et l'éblouissement
à sentir enfin — « agir, je viens ! » — l'action, oui, réelle
(encore au retour dans les rues, etc.)
du déroulement de phrases

que la poésie,
active-décomposante,
plus immédiatement effective que toute assignation à soi,
pouvait délivrer ?

et de pareils anciens instants auront-ils été
une des conditions de possibilité
de mon attention,
si tard, en fin de ma vie,
à la réalité — massive mais suspendue —
de l'existence de K. ?

*

il a voulu revenir mourir chez vous me dit l'ami sénégalais Samba
puis-je le croire ?

si pauvre certitude-larmes

*

nous ne l'aurons pas eue, cette conversation que j'attendais …

non pas seulement celle, si familière, au jour le jour et sans fin, qui avait été la nôtre huit années durant, et que nous aurions naturellement reprise à partir de ce dimanche 15 mars avant de la poursuivre dans les jours et semaines et mois et années qui auraient dû suivre

mais une autre encore, supplémentaire,
plus délibérée naïvement studieuse

celle par laquelle Khaled m'aurait en des endroits cruciaux guidé

> *comme il l'avait fait quelquefois au bord de la Loire :*
> *nous cherchions les endroits où il avait dormi sur les berges de la Loire,*
> *sous ce pont de chemin de fer où une nuit deux de ses amis furent écrasés*

dans le retour
que je voulais entamer

et à laquelle je devrai m'acharner dans les mois qui viennent,
mais désormais
« tout seul »

il ne me sera pas donné de recourir à Khaled
(le happant au passage, à un des moments où il traversait la maison ou le jardin en sifflotant)

NOTES

je ne recevrai pas l'aide — et les vitales difficultés — de paroles qu'il aurait dites en plus,
ou de ses silences,
pour rouvrir ce que j'ai donc noté de tant de minutes partagées, de tant de paroles échangées
huit années durant

*

deux voix
comme jadis sous le coup
du délire de ma mère

deux sources tremblant égales inégales
est-ce là ce qu'il va me falloir réaliser ?

au prix d'irritants tâtonnements
typographiques
(caractères ou corps, « polices »,
« justifications »)

*

si chacune des deux voix devait venir s'écrire réellement
la sienne n'étant il est vrai que celle que je lui attribue
mais la mienne n'ayant lieu que grâce à ce qu'elle aura reçu de la sienne

ce serait en ré-imaginant le suspens créé par l'autre

*

voix, vraiment, prises à ces lignes ?
elles y grésilleraient y tressauteraient
ne cessant de se différencier d'elles-mêmes

il leur faudrait inscrire ici
en variations fiévreuses

leur point d'émission, ou la direction de leur provenance,
ou leur distance (très loin-tout près)
ou leurs multiples vitesses

sans que puissent pourtant se réaliser
les différences d'accent
(d'inclusion ancienne ou récente à la langue française)
ou bien sûr
les singularités matérielles

ultra-sensibles
des voix
— de celle de Khaled

*

voix qui ne devront s'inscrire dans des lignes à former demain
qu'en y ré-imposant — selon quelle brute effectuation ? —

l'espace-temps informe des migrations
qui s'engouffrait entre nous, là, dans la cuisine, quand nous parlions

poignées de pluie et sables tempêtes de haine rouge
averses de vies-morts incomptables
criblant rouges dans la cuisine la parole et l'écoute

*

« **à la maison !** » *s'écria joyeusement Khaled*
alors que, quelques mois après son arrivée dans cette maison,
nous revenions en voiture d'un « rama » quelconque
(un de ces « rama » — Brico, Casto, Confo —
que nous disions « de merde »)
de la banlieue d'Orléans

cette vaste maison séculaire
(qui avait échappé de peu — le hasard de quelque cent mètres —
aux bombardements de 1940 et de 1944
…je lui avais raconté cette histoire)
avait depuis une bonne quarantaine d'années
reçu pour quelques jours ou des mois ou des années
nombre d'« étrangers »

lui seul pourtant
sut la vivre, la sentir, la différencier intérieurement :
murs et sols
volumes de natures distinctes
odeurs-saveurs ou bruits

NOTES

*

à la maison !

Nuruddin Farah, *Hier, demain, voix et témoignages de la diaspora somalienne*, 2000.

Début de l'Avant-propos :

Je suis somalien ; la crise politique somalienne m'a emporté dans son tourbillon au début de l'année 1991, peu après l'effondrement de Mogadiscio. J'habitais non loin de là, à Kampala, en Ouganda ; j'enseignais la littérature à l'Université de Makerere. Je me rappelle avoir pris l'avion pour Nairobi, avant de recevoir un coup de fil très urgent de ma famille proche.

Plus loin, Farah oppose les réfugiés de Mombasa (les pauvres) à ceux de Nairobi (riches et pillards)…

À Mombasa, les réfugiés étaient obsédés par des souvenirs fantomatiques : ils se rappelaient les grenades, les cadavres abandonnés qui pourrissaient aux confins de la capitale. J'étais abattu et comprenais enfin le sens réel du dicton somali selon lequel le souverain bien, c'est d'être propriétaire de sa maison, car on peut jouir alors d'une plus grande intimité, mais aussi garder estime de soi et dignité. Mon père, mon fils, une de mes sœurs cadettes et un de mes neveux étaient arrivés parmi les premiers dans cette cité côtière, et ils devaient partager leur chambre avec de parfaits inconnus. Je me rappelle les propos de ma sœur : « Une maison vous protège, garde vos secrets, veille telle une sentinelle sur votre amour-propre. Peut-être est-ce quand on ne possède pas de maison et qu'on vit dans un pays où ne règne pas la paix qu'on devient réfugié. »

*

l'opacité dans la maison se mouvant sans repos en plein jour
là où est ravalé, remâché, recraché au dehors de l'individuation, de l'avoir à être soi, chaque jour-nuit de la restitution opaque et du réarrachement à une même masse de pouvoir-vivre réaliment des soi distincts

comment devint-elle substantielle exposition-accueil aux interruptions ?

*

c'est dans cette masse durablement vitale « ordinaire » pour quelques vies
que furent possibles
nombre d'irruptions
(depuis la Côte d'Ivoire, les États-Unis, d'Iran, du Cambodge, du Japon, de Chine, de Corée, du Soudan)

                                                               « irruptions » ?
                                                        je cherche des mots —
                          dans les informations, chez les sociologues, les spécialistes
                                                faudrait-il un registre spécifique ?

                         réfugiés, intrusion, hotspots: le nouveau lexique des migrations
                                       10 août 2015 | Par Carine Fouteau (Mediapart) :

                        « Les mots caractérisant les phénomènes migratoires apparaissent ces
                        derniers mois investis de nouvelles significations. Relayés dans l'espace
                        public, ils alimentent les peurs, fabriquent de l'exclusion et confortent
                        l'approche sécuritaire privilégiée par les autorités européennes. »

ou plutôt
des interruptions (dans la vitale continuité familiale)…
et intersections

ou au fil du temps
des inclusions *complexes, imprévues, clignant doucement*
des imbrications *entre existences*

*

or c'est avec Khaled seul — et ce fut pour une part en la recevant de lui, de sa manière d'être —
que l'impulsion me vint et se maintint (obstinée, voire féroce, jour après jour, huit années durant)
de noter

*

dès les premiers temps, presque toujours dans la cuisine ouverte sur le jardin,
je voulus — et bientôt il voulut —
parler, obstinément

au prix de maints petits malentendus (il ne parlait que très peu le français, nous recourions aussi à un peu d'anglais — et à des gestes ou, sur un bout de papier, à des dessins),
de cahots

en revanche, après quelques tentatives,
je renonçai à rien noter sur le champ, sous ses yeux, de ses propos

il me fallait être clairement (sensiblement pour lui comme pour moi) libre de m'absorber dans l'écoute

*

> qu'est-ce donc que noter ?
> une décision... non sans violence ? brutalité ?
>
> noter comme j'allais le faire, huit années durant,
> après avoir écouté Khaled
> m'aurait-il été impossible — voire interdit — pour
> mes enfants ?
>
> à eux, me suis-je dit un jour, j'aurai
> (responsabilité-irresponsabilité béante)
> donné — contribué à donner — **la vie**
>
> Khaled, j'aurais voulu l'aider, de côté (et finalement, en vain),
> à avoir enfin,
> ou de nouveau,
> **...une vie**

*

je recopie ici un passage que j'avais fixé (pour une publication dans un numéro de *Poé&sie*) de nos conversations et où, à sa demande (par crainte de quoi ?), il était nommé Ousmane (ou O.) :

> Noter ce que dit O., depuis bientôt un an qu'il habite ici et qu'il vient régulièrement parler — dans la cuisine, en fin d'après-midi —, j'ai scrupule à le faire pendant qu'il parle. Il hésite, il se heurte moins à des manques de vocabulaire ou aux défaillances de sa syntaxe qu'à sa rugueuse prononciation. Et puis soudain, ses phrases se bousculent, et voici que, sur la table encombrée (journaux, légumes, miettes), je ne trouve pas de papier ; j'attrape un bout de journal, ou une enveloppe déchirée, un crayon qui traîne — pour ne griffonner que mal, de côté, à la dérobée, gêné.
>
> Et puis je répugne à l'interrompre. Ne faudrait-il pas, pourtant, reprononcer ses mots, ou lui retourner, recomposées, ses phrases ?

*

O. s'interrompt souvent lui-même, visage tourné vers le sol.
S'il relève soudain les yeux, je suis gêné d'être surpris à le regarder trop attentivement. Et que penserait-il s'il avait accès à des phrases qui, comme celles-ci, le décrivent ?

Il gratte de l'index le cadre en bois — grossier vernis qui pèle, fibres de pin — de la table (le plateau est de métal émaillé : mode d'il y a bien trente ans).

Bruits, alors, arrivant à travers les vitres — variant selon l'heure du jour ou la saison. Vent, clochette au coin du toit bas de la cuisine… Ou, par la porte entr'ouverte sur le jardin, cris d'aiguilles de mésanges… Ou…

Mais qu'est-ce qui, émanant de son existence si longtemps quasi muette comme de la mienne souvent verbeuse, s'épaissit au-dessus de la table, entre nos visages ? De l'impuissance double, redoublée.

*

… donc : ne jamais noter sur le champ …

avoir d'abord simplement été libre de donner son attention sans projet ou calcul, sans savoir ce qui vous reviendra de ce don (seulement selon la générosité — le bonheur intrinsèque — de l'attention)

ne (re)former des phrases que le lendemain pour me donner le temps de « comprendre » ce que j'aurai entendu ?

prendre le temps, plutôt, que
tout l'entendu de la veille se trouve baigné de sommeil
ou plutôt soit restitué par les rêves
aux boues mouvantes des appartenances,
aux mâchoires archaïques des dépendances féroces

*

aurai-je aube après aube *reformulé* les propos de K. ?
inévitablement, quoique de moins en moins, au fil du temps, son français s'enrichissant…

mais aussi il y avait à essayer de re-capter, en même temps que les paroles et que l'écoute, leur élément propre, la réalité pâle, dans la cuisine, de l'entre…

*

NOTES

> *reconstituer* avant le jour les propos de Khaled de la veille
> m'a paru par instants ressembler à
> **traduire** un poème...
>
> la chose déjà dite par un autre
> la restituer à l'état
> d'une nuée de traits, de possibles grésillants,
> un essaim orageux
> se décomposant-recomposant en l'air
> dans l'entre vies et voix,
> avant de se redéposer frais brûlant
> sur la page, ou l'écran

*

Khaled a glissé du canapé où il était assis, il s'est effondré sur le sol alors même que j'essayais de le rattraper dans mes bras

le 15 mars à 11 heures

sa tête, yeux révulsés, pesait dans ma main ; j'ai senti sa salive s'écouler

je l'ai quitté quelques secondes — pour crier dans la cage d'escalier (vers les amis, Jinjia, Aya, vers Hélène)

je suis revenu à ce corps gisant sur le sol, et le soulevant, et pleurant

(et puis très vite les pompiers, brusques d'abord : « Vous êtes qui pour lui ? », puis le SAMU, un dimanche matin, un médecin, noir par hasard, et soudain parlant, lui, avec précautions et douceur : « c'est très mauvais... » « le cœur »)

(il est mort après trois jours de soins donnés par une équipe qui fut toute d'attention pour lui, pour ce corps que n'animaient plus que des impulsions artificielles, et en même temps, de surcroît, envers nous, prenant du temps pour nous, hébétés, ou pour les amis Soudanais, pour Youssef qui se chargea de téléphoner à sa mère à Khartoum)

*

il y a ces jours-ci (début août 2015) un peu plus de huit ans
depuis qu'avec son ami Hamid, qui traduisait, nous sommes venus jusqu'à ce studio —
dans notre maison dont bientôt il aurait toutes les clés)
et qu'alors je lui ai ouvert
je lui ai dit (fait dire) qu'il pouvait désormais habiter là

il a répondu, par l'intermédiaire de Hamid : je peux pas payer l'eau, pas payer l'électricité

j'ai dit : bien sûr
les yeux me brûlaient — et je voyais les siens briller de larmes

des années plus tard, il me dira : « j'avais peur de pas dire les bons mots »

*

Et comme ça, je n'ai pas répondu à ton appel, je n'ai pas frappé à ta porte ?... mais toi, toi m'as-tu appelé, vraiment ?... et tu m'aurais ouvert la porte, vraiment ?... Et tout le monde peut dire : je n'avais pas d'autre voie et là j'ai rencontré qui j'ai pu !...

De Signoribus, *Ronde des convers : 1999–2004*

*

la poésie De Signoribus

*évidences furtives de gestes référentiels aussitôt évanouis
dans l'obscurité*

*on aura senti leur précision… choses et événements furent certainement là, à portée…
et aussitôt : suspens, dérobement…*

*le poème aura-t-il renoncé à se charger d'informations, d'explicitations référentielles,
documentaires ?*

*c'est plutôt qu'il s'y est instantanément brûlé
il n'y a plus que gestes filaments se rétractant
(et de minuscules échos de cris qui rougeoient se calcinent)*

*

NOTES

bien sûr, Khaled savait que je « notais »

une fois, il m'entendit lire quelques-unes de ces notes, lors d'une « rencontre » à la Maison de la Poésie, un samedi après-midi...
(il était alors à Paris
je ne lui avais pas proposé de venir, nous nous étions vus juste avant dans un café de la rue Beaubourg,
et c'est au sortir de la lecture que j'avais découvert qu'il y avait assisté)

tu prends mes mots, avait-il dit, au retour, à Orléans,
(lentement comme toujours, cherchant ses mots),
tu mets des mots à toi,
tu trouves les bons mots

*

ai-je cru voulu croire une seconde ce 10 août 2015 10h16 que le craquement dans le couloir c'était son pas et qu'il allait arriver subrepticement, ironiquement... pour feindre de me surprendre devant l'ordinateur... et puis éclater de rire ?

*

brusquement, il lui arrivait de survenir
dans cette pièce alors que
je m'évertuais
à reprendre des notes de notre conversation de la veille

brûlant de recréer
pour ses phrases ou les miennes
(celles mêmes qui, la veille, n'avaient cessé de s'écraser
contre d'invisibles obstacles)

de l'élément vital
où elles pourraient ne plus cesser de respirer

branchies de phrases libres sensitives aux filets sanglants déployés

*

il n'y aura pas eu de « parce que c'était lui parce que c'était moi »

nous ne nous étions évidemment pas choisis

la seule brutalité du réel (au départ : la catastrophe au Darfour, puis la Libye, puis …)
l'aura jeté
dans cette maison
en juillet 2007

sa vie démunie plaquée
comme d'une gifle de houle contre nos vies protégées

sur et entre nos vies continues sa vie interrompue

et pourtant celui qui (émergeant de l'anonymisation monstrueuse des migrants)
vécut ici — ce fut, « chez nous »,

lui

*

nous ? famille, maison …

quels qu'en aient été, des années durant, les troubles (doutes, dettes ou coûts réciproques,
cruautés vitales)

**un minimum de cohérence, de continuité,
un fond de constance**

telle fut la condition
pour vivre, pour croire, ou plutôt pour oser **réaliser**
— de notre part
ou de la sienne
cette vie « avec K. »

NOTES

je l'ai senti
au fil des semaines, mois, années
devenir sûr
qu'il pourrait indéfiniment compter sur nous,
sur la maison

*

la constance, certes,
la continuité, oui

mais — et contradictoirement ? —
sans renoncer à défaire de lui-même
l'opaque tenir-à-soi des vies qui se veulent
ou se croient
ordinaires

ou, par impossible,
sans trop contribuer au mensonge toujours réitéré
— dans ses obtuses promesses à elle-même —
de la « vie douce »

celle dont j'aurai tenté depuis des années
de dérouler, de côté,
les douteuses évidences

sans jamais consentir à la version dévorante (destructrice de possibles)
de la cohérence

sans (s'il se pouvait) participer de la férocité de tant de vies voulant se croire « chez elles »

celles qui ne vivent leur « ordinaire » et leur adhésion à elles-mêmes
qu'au prix de dénier les surgissements non prévus
naissant en et de leur obscure « intimité » même

celles qui projettent leurs propres ruptures internes
(les bords acérés qui se forment irrésistiblement en elles, entre elles, par elles)
pour les changer en violence et cruauté « hors »
contre de prétendument tout autres

*

c'est pour Khaled le premier, ce fut quasiment pour lui seul,

après Ibrahim-Kim-Pedram-Farzam-Laura
ou, tout autrement, certes mais non sans interactions,
Linda
ou
Masatsugu, Jinjia, Aya, Méï...

(cette énumération boite-blesse :
— tant de singularités !
et pour les quatre derniers de liens avec Khaled)

et presque dès son arrivée ici,
que l'évidence s'imposa, impérative aveuglante, qu'il fallait noter

fut-ce du fait qu'il venait du Darfour, dont il avait fui les violences génocidaires ?

de celles auxquelles, depuis des années,
comme pas mal d'autres intellectuels des récentes décennies,
j'avais appris à prêter
une attention spéciale
— éthico-politique ? voire poético-politique : afin de **réaliser** ? —
mais qui devait-devrait ne pas cesser d'être elle-même
l'objet d'une inquiétude critique
(n'était-ce pas dès alors ce « mal de vérité » que travaille Catherine Coquio ?)

d'autres cependant — Kim (les Khmers rouges), Pedram, Farzam (l'Iran, la guerre Iran-Irak), Laura (l'Angola) — avaient fui des violences extrêmes —

quel changement spécifique se fit lors de l'arrivée de Khaled dans mon double désir de ne pas seulement écouter, mais de quotidiennement m'évertuer à former-formuler ?

*

j'avais jusqu'alors (sans y penser)
cloisonné

il m'avait fallu maintenir
entre deux régions d'existence
— celle des présences-irruptions (ou de la multiforme disponibilité et de l'inventivité qu'elles
requéraient : pour l'écoute ou pour maints soucis de vie)
et, tout près, tout autre
celle de mes tentatives « propres » (lire-écrire, évidemment, etc.)

j'avais œuvré à la condition de possibilité de tout le reste :
une stricte **séparation**... jamais pensée,
simplement incarnée dans cette maison même, ses volumes ou temps internes
j'avais créé maintenu obscurément obstinément

une étanchéité

*

> *à l'endroit*
> *le plus réceptif*
> *se dresse le mur qui se bâtit*
> *lui-même, et cela de telle façon*
> *qu'il ne pouvait autrement*
>
> Vladimir Holan, « *Le mur qui se bâtit lui-même* »

*

**Or Khaled lui aussi
cloisonnait**

> dans les trois jours entre l'effondrement chez nous de Khaled et sa mort à l'hôpital,
> puis dans les semaines qui suivirent, et aujourd'hui encore,
> des Soudanais, venant d'Orléans ou de Paris ou d'autres villes — Lyon —,
> ont manifesté leur attention
> et leur désir de proximité

> j'avais rencontré un certain nombre d'entre eux, sinon tous,
> chez Khaled, dans son studio
> mais c'était toujours brièvement
> — par discrétion de ma part (ce que Khaled, parfois, humoristiquement, me reprochait : « tu restes jamais... »),

        mais aussi, comme me l'a expliqué l'un des amis, Youssef, du fait que Khaled tenait clairement
                (au moins à certains moments et sur certains points)
        à ne pas laisser s'imposer dans notre maison un excès d'afflux

            …quelques semaines après la mort de Khaled,
    Jinjia, l'ami chinois (du premier étage de la maison), alors que revenant ensemble de Paris,
            nous conversons dans le train de nuit,
        reprend le terme de « cloisonnement » que je viens d'employer :
                cloisonner, suggère-t-il
            — maintenir des zones d'existence distinctes —
        fut nécessaire à K., au précaire « équilibre » de sa vie-survie

et donc, ai-je appris tardivement à comprendre,
quand nous parlions, c'était lui, là — et pas tout lui

car, ne serait-ce que pour parler dans la cuisine
(et en sachant que j'allais noter),
il lui fallait maintenir des écarts dans les liens mêmes…

des non-franchissements
sans brutalité,
avec délicatesse, humour

mais pour ne pas rendre impossible… quoi ? dans sa vie… ses rapports et liens ?

        ou parfois, comme malgré lui, maintenait-il des parts de solitude
           entre lui et nous entre nous et les autres (Soudanais)
                entre lui et les Soudanais

                    des lames de vide
                    des souffles froids ?

                *

pour moi du moins le cloisonnement
    a cessé insensiblement d'avoir lieu

l'étanchéité entre régions de la vie
dans la cohabitation familiale avec Khaled

ne put comme en un sourire
que céder

un mur mental n'avait plus lieu d'être
consentant à son inutilité, il s'était effondré
en ne soufflant que douceur

une paroi interne du cœur
cuite jour après jour d'attention

mauve brunie et friable

avait dû à mon insu se désagréger :

dissoute
dans l'ombre limpide de l'affection pour Khaled

évanouie

COLOPHON

ENTANGLED — PAPERS! — NOTES

was handset in InDesign CC

The text and page numbers are set in *Adobe Jenson Pro*

The titles are set in *Didonesque Display*.

Book design & typesetting: Alessandro Segalini

Cover design: A. Segalini, C. Mouchard, M. Shaw

Cover image: Paul Klee, *Von der Liste gestrichen (Struck from the List)*, 1933, Zentrum Paul Klee, Bern

Calligraphy: Alessandro Segalini

ENTANGLED — PAPERS! — NOTES

is published by Contra Mundum Press.
Its printer has received Chain of Custody certification from:
The Forest Stewardship Council,
The Programme for the Endorsement of Forest Certification,
& The Sustainable Forestry Initiative.

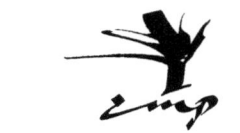

Contra Mundum Press   New York · London · Melbourne

CONTRA MUNDUM PRESS

Dedicated to the value & the indispensable importance of the individual voice, to works that test the boundaries of thought & experience.

The primary aim of Contra Mundum is to publish translations of writers who in their use of form and style are *à rebours*, or who deviate significantly from more programmatic & spurious forms of experimentation. Such writing attests to the volatile nature of modernism. Our preference is for works that have not yet been translated into English, are out of print, or are poorly translated, for writers whose thinking & æsthetics are in opposition to timely or mainstream currents of thought, value systems, or moralities. We also reprint obscure and out-of-print works we consider significant but which have been forgotten, neglected, or overshadowed.

There are many works of fundamental significance to *Weltliteratur* (& *Weltkultur*) that still remain in relative oblivion, works that alter and disrupt standard circuits of thought — these warrant being encountered by the world at large. It is our aim to render them more visible.

For the complete list of forthcoming publications, please visit our website. To be added to our mailing list, send your name & email address to: info@contramundum.net

Contra Mundum Press
P.O. Box 1326
New York, NY 10276
USA

THE MÆCENAS CONSTELLATION

The Mæcenas Constellation (MC) is an alternative patronage experiment composed of individuals who together will form the inner circle of Contra Mundum Press. Through its combined resources, the constellation will serve as an entity akin to a Renaissance patron.

Contra Mundum Press is an award-winning independent publishing house that has published translations from Sumerian, French, Hungarian, Italian, German, Turkish, and Farsi, two world-premiere editions of Pessoa, and several bi- and multilingual books from a variety of genres. Our art journal, *Hyperion: On the Future of Æsthetics*, has an international readership stretching from the Americas to Europe, Africa, the Middle East, and Asia. Writers such as Erika Burkart, Quentin Meillassoux, Alain Badiou, and others have contributed original essays to the journal. Contra Mundum Press has also staged events and collaborated with numerous cultural institutions in New York, Budapest, Berlin, Paris, & elsewhere, including participating in international film and literary festivals. Since our inception in 2012, our publications have been heralded in the pages of *The Times Literary Supplement*, *The New Statesman*, *The Guardian*, the *Paris Review*, and the *Los Angeles Review of Books*, amongst others. To become a member of the Mæcenas Constellation is to express your confidence in and support of such cultural work, and to aid us in continuing it.

Becoming a member of the MC simply involves a modest pledge of only $60 per year. The funds received from such a membership body would not only help compensate for the bulk of the production costs of producing six books per year, it would also provide some financial support for the different experiences the collective wishes to develop. Aside from receiving 2 books per year in advance of publication and a limited edition tote bag, you would be entitled to a 30% discount when purchasing any of our other books (which you would receive in advance of release to the general public). Additionally, you will be offered the opportunity of purchasing limited edition books only available to members.

Through our community of readers, we would then be able to remain an independent entity free of having to rely on government support and/or grant and other official funding bodies, not to speak of their timelines & impositions. It would also free the press from suffering the vagaries of the publishing industry, as well as the risk of submitting to commercial pressures in order to persist, thereby potentially compromising the integrity of its catalog.

With bookstores and presses around the world struggling to survive, and many even closing, we hope to establish this alternative form of patronage as a means for establishing a continuous & stable foundation to safeguard the longevity of Contra Mundum Press. Each individual member of the constellation would help to form a greater entity and so jointly advance the cultural efforts of Contra Mundum Press. A unified assemblage of individuals can make a modern Mæcenas.

To lend your support and BECOME A MEMBER, please visit the subscription page of our website: *contramundum.net/subscription*

OTHER CONTRA MUNDUM PRESS TITLES

Gilgamesh
Ghérasim Luca, *Self-Shadowing Prey*
Rainer J. Hanshe, *The Abdication*
Walter Jackson Bate, *Negative Capability*
Miklós Szentkuthy, *Marginalia on Casanova*
Fernando Pessoa, *Philosophical Essays*
Elio Petri, *Writings on Cinema & Life*
Friedrich Nietzsche, *The Greek Music Drama*
Richard Foreman, *Plays with Films*
Louis-Auguste Blanqui, *Eternity by the Stars*
Miklós Szentkuthy, *Towards the One & Only Metaphor*
Josef Winkler, *When the Time Comes*
William Wordsworth, *Fragments*
Josef Winkler, *Natura Morta*
Fernando Pessoa, *The Transformation Book*
Emilio Villa, *The Selected Poetry of Emilio Villa*
Robert Kelly, *A Voice Full of Cities*
Pier Paolo Pasolini, *The Divine Mimesis*
Miklós Szentkuthy, *Prae, Vol. 1*
Federico Fellini, *Making a Film*
Robert Musil, *Thought Flights*
Sándor Tar, *Our Street*
Lorand Gaspar, *Earth Absolute*
Josef Winkler, *The Graveyard of Bitter Oranges*
Ferit Edgü, *Noone*
Jean-Jacques Rousseau, *Narcissus*
Ahmad Shamlu, *Born Upon the Dark Spear*
Jean-Luc Godard, *Phrases*
Otto Dix, *Letters, Vol. 1*
Maura Del Serra, *Ladder of Oaths*
Pierre Senges, *The Major Refutation*
Charles Baudelaire, *My Heart Laid Bare & Other Texts*
Joseph Kessel, *Army of Shadows*
Rainer J. Hanshe, *Shattering the Muses*
Gerard Depardieu, *Innocent*

SOME FORTHCOMING TITLES

Pierre Senges, *Ahab (Sequels)*
Gœthe, *The Passion of Young Werther*

ABOUT THE AUTHOR

Claude Mouchard is a poet and translator, emeritus professor of Comparative Literature at Université Paris 8 — Saint-Denis, and associate editor-in-chief of *Po&sie*, one of France's leading poetry journals. He is the author of many critical works, including *Un grand désert d'hommes, 1851–1885. Les équivoques de la modernité* (1991) and *Qui si je criais…? Œuvres-témoignages dans les tourmentes du XXᵉ siècle* (2007), a wide-ranging reflection on testimonial works born of 20th-century political catastrophes. He has published three collections of poetry (*Ici*, 1986; *Perdre*, 1979 and 1989; *L'Air*, 1997), the "pamphlet poem" *Papiers!* (2007), and several series of what he simply calls *Notes*, whose experimental language focuses on the plight of the exiled and homeless in France. He is currently completing a critical volume on Korean poetry, *Voix de Corée*, and three poetic works: *La vie douce*, *Avec Khaled*, and *Rafales Grünewald*. *Entangled — Papers! — Notes*, a bilingual edition of selected works, offers the first English translation of Claude Mouchard's poetry.

ABOUT THE TRANSLATOR

Mary Shaw is a poet and professor of French Literature at Rutgers University — New Brunswick. Along with such critical works as *Performance in the Texts of Mallarmé* (1993), *The Cambridge Introduction to French Poetry* (2003), and *Visible Writings: Forms, Cultures, Readings* (co-edited with Marija Dalbello, 2011), she has published two children's books and a collection of poems, *Album Without Pictures* (2008). Her *dreamscapes* regularly appear in the online journal *Transitions*, and have also been published in *Hyperion: The Future of Æsthetics* (2017) as a series entitled "A Mallarmé Fan Suite," as well as in the journals *Po&sie* (2015) and *Versants* (2015) in French translations. She is currently working on gathering a first volume of these texts, to be entitled *dreamscapes — 100 nights*.

www.ingramcontent.com/pod-product-compliance
Lightning Source LLC
Chambersburg PA
CBHW081126170426
43197CB00017B/2769